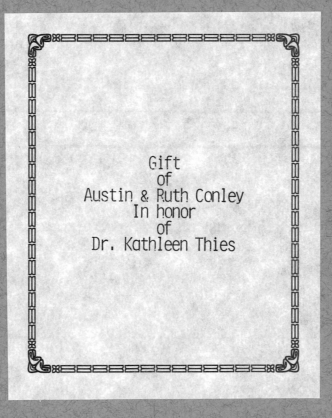

Gift
of
Austin & Ruth Conley
In honor
of
Dr. Kathleen Thies

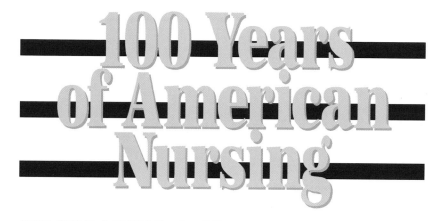

100 Years of American Nursing

CELEBRATING A CENTURY OF CARING

100 Years of American Nursing

CELEBRATING A CENTURY OF CARING

Thelma M. Schorr, BSN, RN, FAAN

Former Editor, *American Journal of Nursing*; Former President and Publisher, American Journal of Nursing Company

With

Maureen Shawn Kennedy, MA, RN

Education Specialist/Director, Special Programs, Lippincott Williams & Wilkins

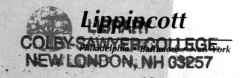

Lippincott

Philadelphia • Baltimore • New York

#4068169l

Acquisitions Editor: Susan M. Glover, RN, MSN
Editorial Assistant: Bridget Blatteau
Senior Project Editor: Erika Kors
Senior Production Manager: Helen Ewan
Senior Production Coordinator: Michael Carcel
Designer: Doug Smock
Cover Illustration: Neal Hughes

9   8   7   6   5   4   3   2   1

Library of Congress Cataloging-in-Publication Data
Schorr, Thelma M.
        100 years of American nursing/Celebrating a century of caring
    Thelma M. Schorr with Maureen Shawn Kennedy.
            p.   cm.
        Includes bibliographical references.
        ISBN 0-7817-1865-1 (alk. paper)
        1. Nursing—United States—History.   I. Kennedy, Maureen Shawn,
    1949–   .   II.   Title.
        [DNLM: 1. History of Nursing—United States.   WY 11 AA1 S374c 1999]
    RT4.S375   1999
    610.73′0973—dc21
    DNLM/DLC
    for Library of Congress   99-10472
                                                                                     CIP

Care has been taken to confirm the accuracy of the information presented and to describe generally accepted practices. However, the authors, editors, and publisher are not responsible for errors or omissions or for any consequences from application of the information in this book and make no warranty, express or implied, with respect to the contents of the publication.

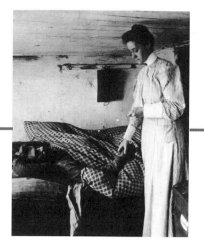

Foreword

From its very first article by the superintendent of nurses on the hospital ship *Maine* on its way to care for casualties in the Boer War in 1900, the *American Journal of Nursing* has chronicled the wonderful and terrible, brilliant and dull, exciting and nondescript, uplifting and depressing strands out of which are woven the tapestry of 100 years of American nursing.

This book is a testament to all the nurses whose experiences have become the history of nursing in America. Yet it is not a history book but rather an impressionistic and photographic study of the profession, told by its members and set against the epic events that have characterized each decade—wars, epidemics, social upheaval, earthquakes, the development of antibiotics, space missions, civil unrest and human rights victories. The pictures illustrate the story of nurses who have struggled throughout the century to improve their education, to enrich their caring practices, and to advance the status of the profession and the reach of its influence. To probe these efforts, we invited 16 well-known and highly respected nursing leaders to present commentaries on a variety of issues, past and present.

We offered the caveat that this is not a history book. Researching it, however, has been an incredibly pleasurable historical adventure. We hope that it will spark historical interest in many of you and will send you each into the early volumes—and the later ones, too—so that you can revel with us in the remarkable history nurses have built in this century.

Thelma M. Schorr
Maureen Shawn Kennedy

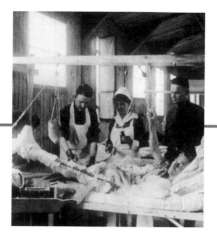

The Journal*'s Editors*

SOPHIA F. PALMER

"We stand today united in the belief that 'State registration' is necessary for our progress; that without it we remain stationary; retrogression, under these circumstances, being the inevitable result . . . . We are not working for ourselves in this matter, but for those who are to come after us . . . ."
DECEMBER 1901

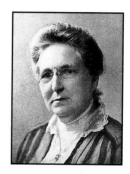

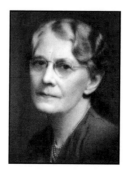

MARY M. ROBERTS

". . . each generation of nurses must live within the framework of its own times. Many of those who have won greatest honor in nursing have no academic degrees. But with changing times, degrees are becoming a commonplace. There is no magic in them . . . . It is only when they represent knowledge which can be put to use in specific situations that they have importance in nursing."
APRIL 1933

NELL V. BEEBY

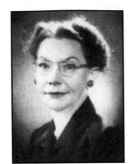

"Respect for the personality of individuals—of every individual—is one of the basic concepts of democracy. . . . Acceptance of this principle is essential to success in any of the various types of teamwork which are currently being described in . . . this magazine for the patient is the focal point of all our efforts."
APRIL 1949

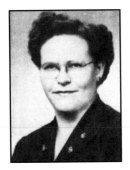

JEANETTE V. WHITE

"Perhaps 'a rose is a rose is a rose,' but a nurse is much more than a nurse . . . each of us must realize that she—or he—is more than a nurse. We may identify ourselves as nurses first; that is understandable. But we are also citizens, members of the community, of religious groups, and many others to which we are obligated."
OCTOBER 1956

EDITH P. LEWIS

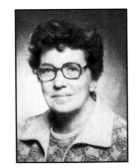

"Nursing has become too big, too important, a profession for us to hope or want to keep our problems to ourselves. It is our right—indeed, our obligation—to correct errors in fact, to express our presumably more informed opinion—in relation to articles about nursing in the popular press."
DECEMBER 1958

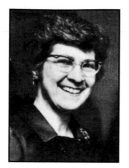

BARBARA G. SCHUTT

"A well-organized, self-governing nursing staff should be as essential to an institution as an organized medical staff. It's time for staff nurses to recognize that they abdicate both collective and individual responsibility when they fail to seek the enforcement of the standards of the nursing profession."
JANUARY 1966

THELMA M. SCHORR

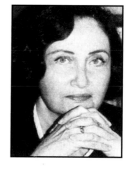

"Medical care is medicine's jargon and it is what most physicians call the total range of health services that patients need. Whether physicians differentiate in their minds that what they are providing is one part of a greater whole, which they call medical care, or whether they see their part as the whole, with all other health professionals providing ancillary services, I don't know.

What I do know is that we in nursing had better recognize how this jargon of theirs is diminishing us and devaluing our contribution to patient care. We had better become much more conscious of the subconscious effect it creates and the stereotype it resurrects.

I am angered by nurses who call themselves "medical personnel" and ignore the implications of their sloppy semantics . . . .

For too long, all health personnel have been lumped under the medical umbrella and as a result, not only we, but the public as well, have been getting drenched."
MAY 1977

MARY B. MALLISON

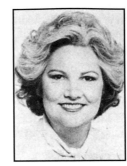

"We've learned to move our observations inside the patient. Thus, 'average' med-surg nurses, not only those in ICUs, follow blood gases and chemistries, draw and measure blood sugars, measure venous pressures and ventilator pressures, track blood cultures, and listen to lung and bowel sounds as well as heart rhythms . . . .

Those who say these functions are medical, not nursing, bury their heads in a romantic nonexistent past. Nurses have always pushed, pulled, and coached patients through their illnesses. Nurses have always made the technology bearable and understandable, have known when to use it more frequently or when to gradually withdraw it. Whether the technology is poultices or ventilators, the nursing attitudes are the same."
MARCH 1988

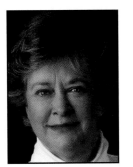

LUCILLE A. JOEL

"If there's a single characteristic that must define the nurse of the '90s, it's the spirit of the intrapreneur working for constructive change, allowing health care institutions to survive financially while still honoring their commitment to the public. Intrapreneurs anticipate what the system needs most—whether it's to cut costs, increase revenue, promote productivity, or shape a new public image.

Intrapreneurs play intelligent hunches, trust their intuition, and thrive on risky business. But they value the security that an organizational affiliation guarantees."
JANUARY 1994

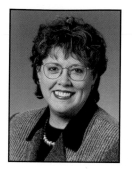

DIANA MASON

"Politics plays a role in every aspect of health care, ranging from what kind of care gets funded to whether a patient gets adequate teaching before being discharged from the hospital. Whereas the politics of health policy are acknowledged and accepted, the politics of bedside care are not so obvious, but hardly less important."
1985

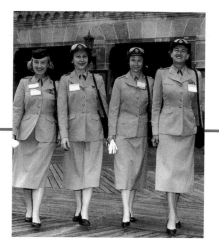

Acknowledgments

We gratefully acknowledge the following individuals who were generous in their time and support: Adele Herwitz, who helped out of her experience on the staffs of the American Nurses Association, the International Council of Nurses, and the Commission on Graduates of Foreign Nursing Schools; historian Shirley Fondiller; Jean Waldman, RN, nurse historian, and Elizabeth Hooks, photo archivist, from the American Red Cross; Major Cynthia Brown, RN, U.S. Army Nurse Corps historian; and Sean Noel from Boston University Special Collections.

MetLife®   We especially thank the Metropolitan Life Insurance Company for their partial sponsorship and applaud them for their continued support of nurses and nursing throughout the years.

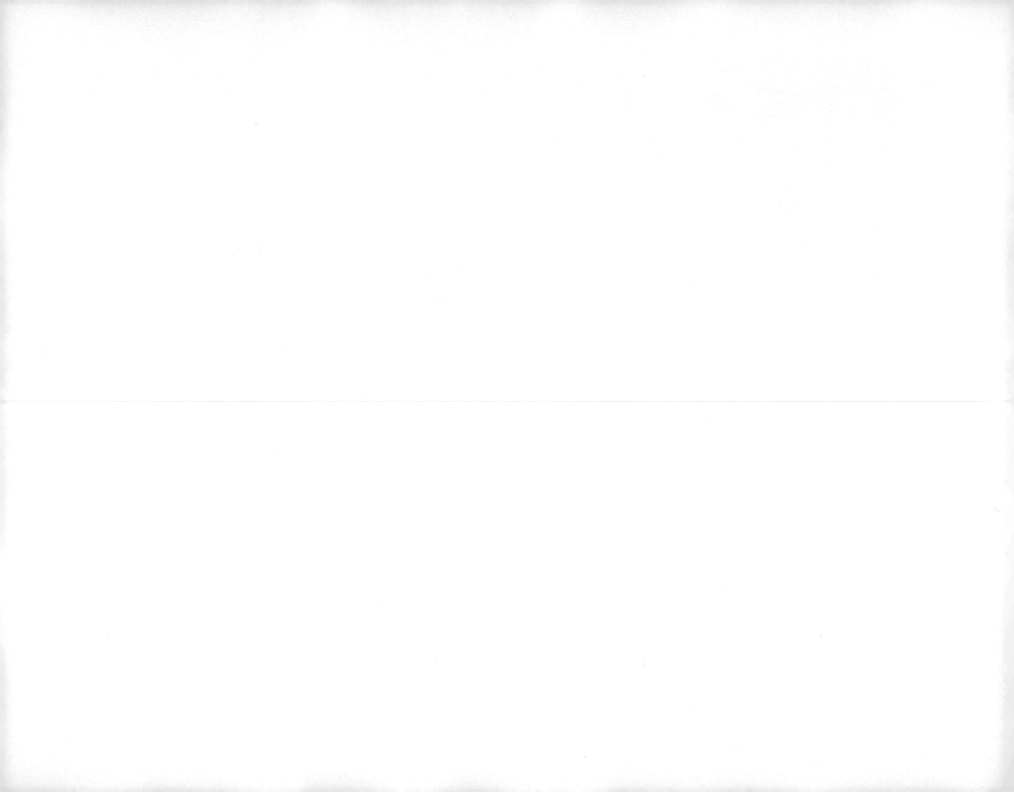

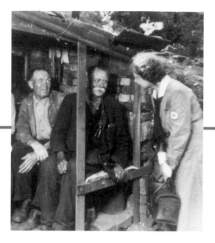

Contents

Photo credits are listed after the index.

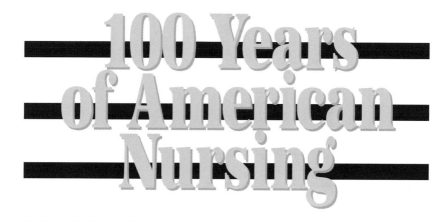

100 Years of American Nursing

CELEBRATING A CENTURY OF CARING

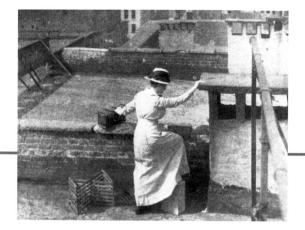

The Early Years

1900–1913

"We are forced to acknowledge the truth of the idea that the world can progress, and nursing can progress, only according to the moral strength and wisdom and courage of its women standing together for what is best for the whole."

So wrote Sophia Palmer, the *American Journal of Nursing*'s first editor, in 1905. And stand together they did, those early nursing giants like Lavinia Dock, Lillian Wald, Isabel Hampton Robb, M. Adelaide Nutting, Linda Richards, Lystra Gretter, Jane Delano, Annie Goodrich, and others like them. They built nursing organizations through which they established registration and fought for standards to give meaning to the term "registered nurse." They struggled against the proliferation of inadequate schools and exploitative short postgraduate courses that used the nurse's service and gave no teaching in return.

At the turn of the century, nurses had few choices when they finished their training. They could work as private duty nurses in patients' homes or in hospitals as superintendents or head nurses, although these opportunities were few. Between cases, private duty nurses lived in boarding houses or nurses' clubs and worried about what they would live on as they grew older. Articles and Letters to the Editor in the early years presented an ongoing debate—should what little money nurses had go into life insurance or bank accounts?

Public health concerns about infant and child care and about infectious diseases, tuberculosis in particular, gave rise to visiting nursing, which ensured that the poor and the middle class received the kind of attention—in small part—that private duty nurses were providing for wealthier patients. Agencies like the Henry Street Settlement in New York City sent nurses into the tenements; nurses in Baltimore's Visiting Nurse Association were employed to follow up tuberculosis patients in their homes; for the rural poor, the Red Cross established a rural nursing service that eventually became the Town and Country Nursing Service, expanding its scope to serve those in small towns as well.

In 1902, Lillian Wald convinced the New York City Board of Education to fund nurses in schools to provide and monitor children's health care. She proved her point by sending one of the Henry Street nurses, Lina Rogers, to do a one-month school nursing project that proved an unqualified success. In June 1909, the amazing Miss Wald, arguing that preventing illness was cheaper than caring for the ill, suggested to the Metropolitan Life Insurance Company that it provide nursing services to policy holders through visiting nurse associations. At the end of 1909 there were 14 Metropolitan visiting nursing services; by 1912 there were 589 throughout the country.

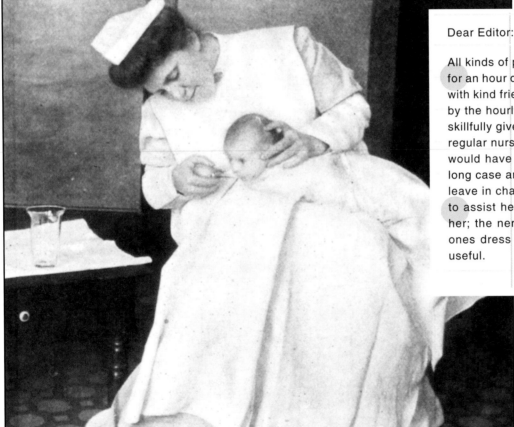

Private duty baby nurse.

Dear Editor:

All kinds of people have found us useful: the doctor who needed a nurse for an hour or two in his office or for a minor operation; the chronic invalid with kind friends to do much for him but whose day and night were eased by the hourly morning and evening visit when the bath and the rub were skillfully given; the woman living in the boardinghouse with no room for a regular nurse and to whom the expense of both the nurse and her board would have been out of the question; the private nurse tired out with a long case and unable to get air and rest without a responsible person to leave in charge; the careful mother with the sick child needing someone to assist her in carrying out the special order that would have agitated her; the nervous, retiring woman, shrinking from having her own loved ones dress the chronic sore. All of these have found the hourly nurse useful.

October 1905

In between cases, most private duty nurses lived in nurses' clubs—their wages would not support a private apartment or home.

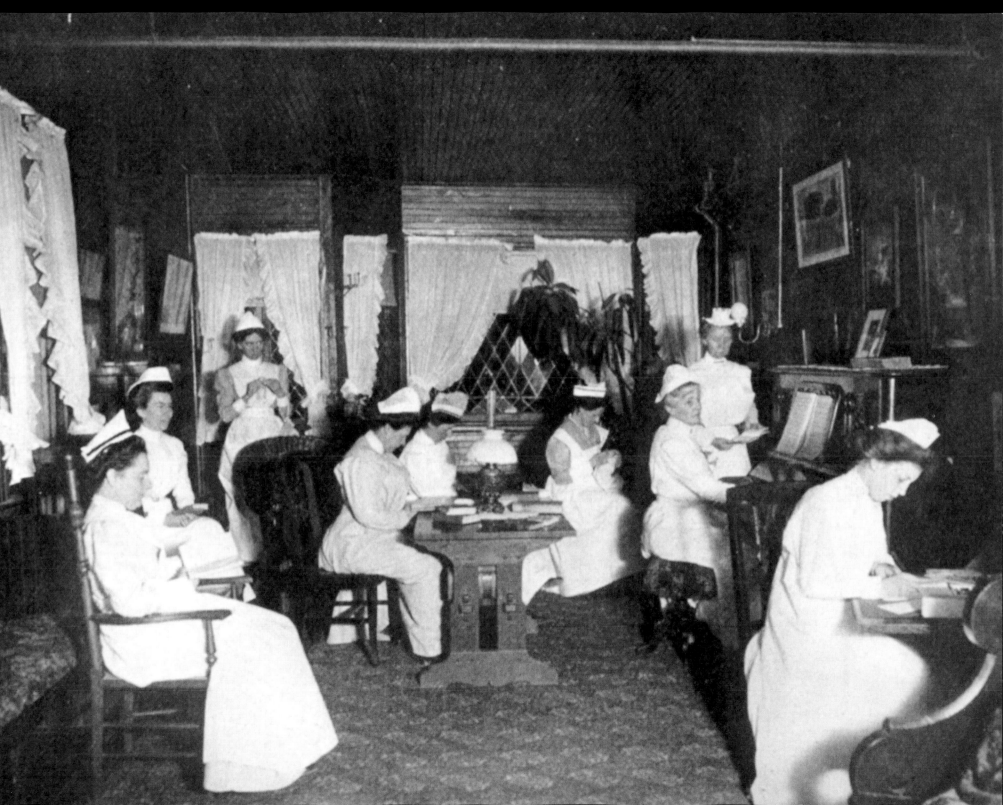

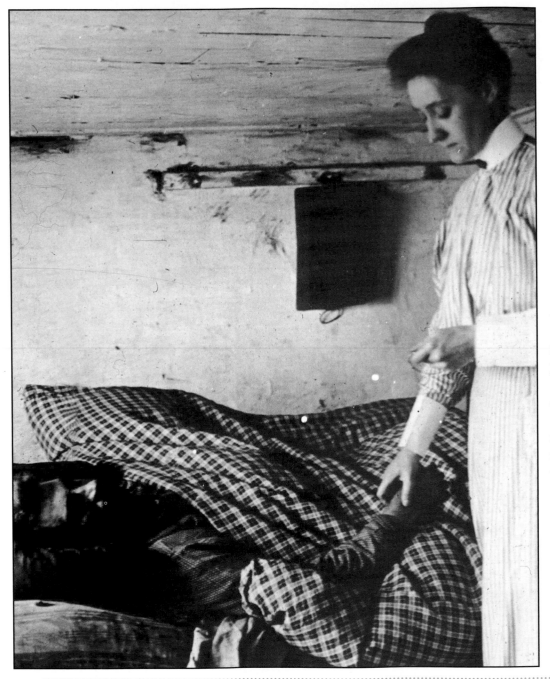

Admonition to a Private Duty Nurse

Never share a bed with your patient may be good advice for some of our newly graduated nurses who start out in private work.

Often one is called to a hotel or a private house where only a little room is at the disposal of you and your patient.

When night comes, the patient, glowing with fever, says frequently: "Miss S., do not sit on that hard chair during the night. Look—this bed is a double one, with room enough for two. Come share it with me, for you need rest. Do please me; it will be a comfort to have you near me."

Now, here comes the temptation to a nurse to please her patient, but stop a moment, think of your patient's and your own welfare.

A patient must have undisturbed rest. Can she have it if the nurse turns or even moves? Does it not annoy a sick person? Is it right for a nurse to allow herself to try to rest with a patient who is restless, coughs, or has fever? Certainly not.

FEBRUARY 1907

Commentary

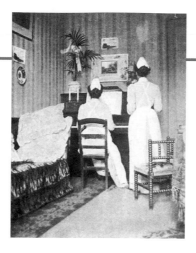

Ellen D. Baer

Private Duty Nursing

Formal training for nurses in the United States began in 1873, with the formation of schools in New York, Connecticut, and Boston. The success of these programs was followed rapidly by the development of training schools in hospitals all over the nation. Each of these hospital schools admitted women for a two-year course of study (later three) that qualified them, upon graduation, to work as trained nurses in the private homes of the sick. Known as private duty nursing, this was the main form of employment for the first fifty years of nursing in America.

Because pupil-nurses performed the nursing work in hospitals, these institutions had no need to hire more than a few supervisory graduate nurses. When public health nursing and visiting nurse associations were established in the 1890s and later, they offered graduate nurses an additional opportunity for paid work and self-sufficiency. But for the large majority of graduate nurses, private duty nursing was the predominant form of available work.

As graduates, private duty nurses found their positions through the recommendations of family physicians, druggists, satisfied former patients, city directories, and nursing agencies. Registries were operated by medical and nursing societies, hospitals, and commercial interests—all with varying standards and requirements. For instance, some hospital nursing programs maintained registries that would recommend graduates only if the graduate was considered "morally sound."

For the most part, private duty nurses went from case to case, living in the homes of their clients for the duration of their responsibility, and otherwise lodging in boarding houses, graduate nurses' clubs, or other such arrangements. In times of sickness, economic recession, or sporadic unemployment, these nurses had no alternative means of support. In many cases, they looked to their colleagues in alumnae associations for financial, social, and political assistance. In 1904, a private duty nurse made $15 per week, from which she had to pay all her own expenses, and on which she could only depend for an average of 33 to 35 weeks per year.

Financial problems continually plagued the private duty nurse. As the reputation of hospitals improved, patients went there more readily for care during illness. As a consequence, private duty nurses expanded their work, agreeing to take on "special" cases in hospitals. Whether working through referrals in private duty or "specialing" a patient in the hospital's private pavilion, most graduate nurses found their fees subject to hospital scrutiny. Difficulties were compounded when certain hospitals emerged as unexpected competitors for nurses' work. Seeking to gain income from the nurses' training school, the Presbyterian Hospital of Philadelphia, for example, sent pupil-nurses into private homes and charged a fee equal to that of the graduate nurse. This positioned the pupil-nurse in unwitting competition with the graduate nurse, although the hospital kept the fees they earned.

As the nation's economic status deteriorated at the end of the 1920s, private duty work for nurses became more and more scarce. Some nurses, led by the American Nurses Association (ANA) director, Janet Geister, tried, without success, to solve the private duty crisis through the creative use of registries as group practices that could supply nurses for many community needs, such as chronic care. Fearing, however, that such activities would be competitive with public health and visiting nursing, the ANA did not pursue this avenue of development.

Although hospital staff nursing replaced private duty work as the major form of employment for graduate nurses after the 1930s, private duty nursing continued to embody many of nursing's ideals regarding one-on-one continuous patient care. The private duty nurse was described as what an ill patient wants most—"someone around constantly who is skilled, can be trusted, and belongs to him."

Most patient care in hospitals was given by students. The few graduate nurses employed by hospitals were in supervisory positions. All other graduates became private duty nurses and, later, visiting nurses or hourly nurses.

Boston Children's Hospital, circa 1905.

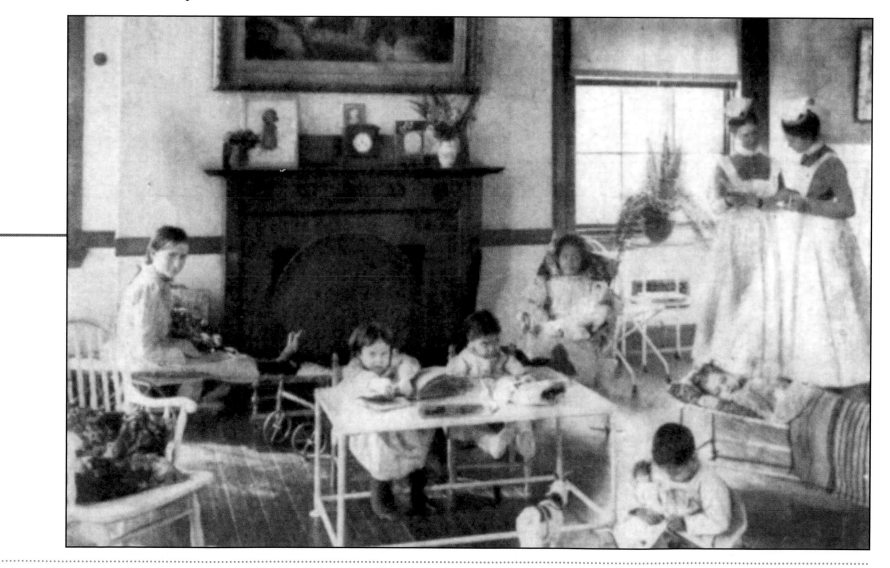

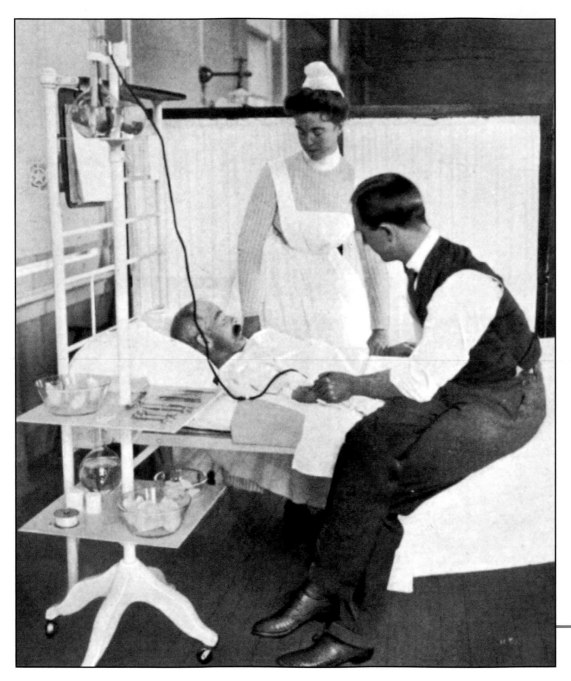

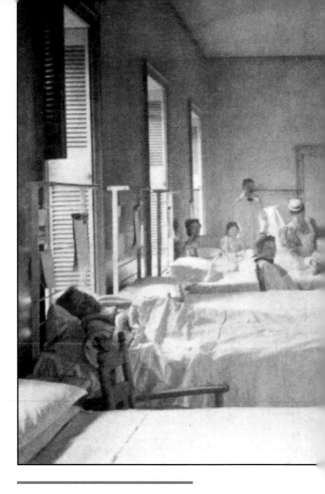

Massachusetts General Hospital.

Hypodermoclysis and saline infusion in the Presbyterian Hospital, New York City.

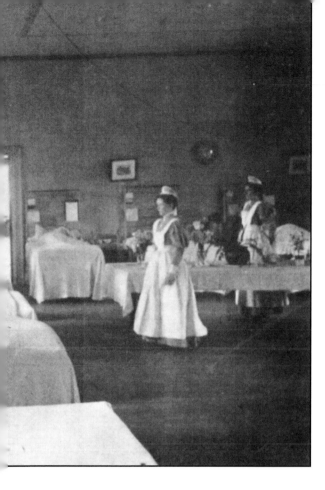

First head nurses at Bellevue, circa 1900.

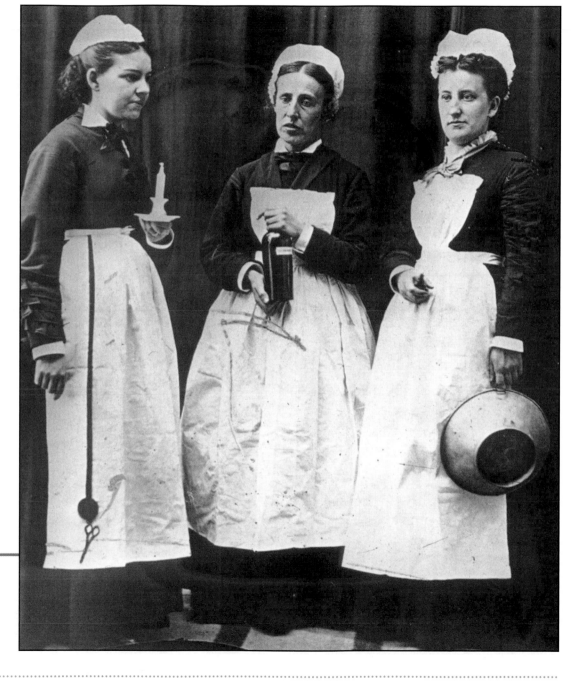

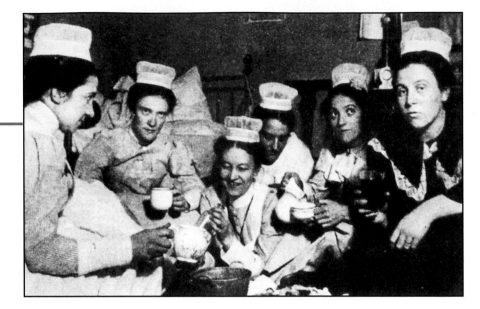

Afternoon tea and midnight feasts seem to be traditional in nursing.

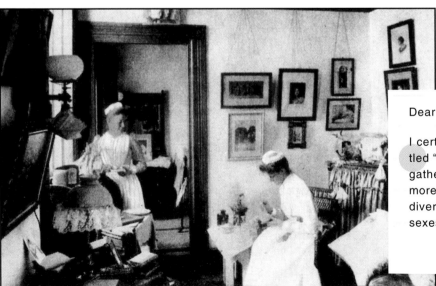

Dear Editor:

I certainly endorse the ideas suggested in your editorial comment entitled "More of the Social." As a class I am sure we do not go in for social gatherings as much as we ought. No class of workers need recreation more than nurses. In nurses' houses it is all business and no play. Surely diversion, and not diversion confined to one sex, but the mingling of sexes, is desirable.

October 1902

The senior nurses of the University of Michigan Training-School, Ann Arbor, Michigan, having finished their class work, have organized themselves into a self-governing study club. Strict parliamentary procedure is practiced. Topics of interest are discussed and occasionally some of the ladies of the city who have had trained nurses in their homes are invited to speak to them.

Some of the subjects which have been drafted for discussion are: "How to Read Aloud," "Etiquette Aside from its Ceremonial Observance," "How to Observe," "The Hygiene of the Sick-Room," "Modes of Preservation of Food," "The So-Called 'Personal Equation.'" The nurses are very enthusiastic, and it is hoped that much beneficial work may be accomplished before the first of September.

JUNE 1901

Students practice on each other in a bandaging lesson.

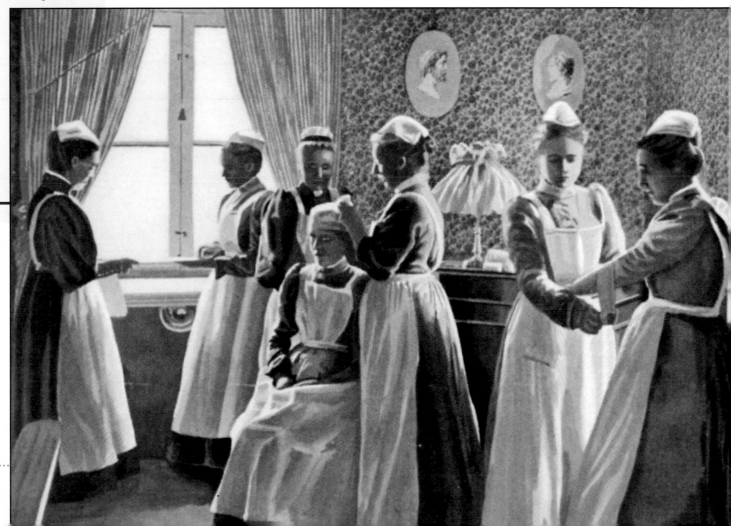

Report from Lillian Wald: THE NURSES' SETTLEMENT IN NEW YORK CITY

The number of patients on the books in the last year was forty-four hundred and seventy-two; nursing visits made, twenty-five thousand eight hundred and forty; first aid cases treated, fifteen thousand five hundred and fourteen.

The settlement has twelve nurses on district duty in different parts of the city, while those in charge of the country home, the town houses, and first aid and supervisory work bring the number to seventeen. Besides these, one nurse more is engaged in teaching and organizing household and home-making classes.

There are also resident a young woman who teaches carpentry and basket making, a young kindergartner, who takes charge of the dancing-classes, and, in the winter, Mrs. Florence Kelly, secretary of the Consumers' League.

In the coming year it is expected that extensions in the nursing service will be made.

The enlargements in the past year were the opening of a summer home for children and young girls, the gift of a new town house, the alteration of one of the old ones as permanent club quarters, and the renting of a small house for the carpentry classes.

FEBRUARY 1902

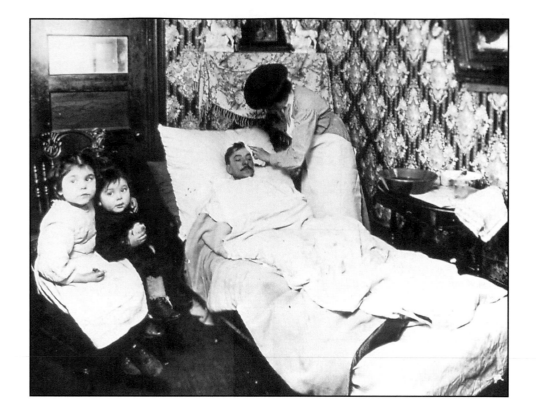

After the downfall of Tammany the public press commented to some extent upon the work of the "Settlements" as a factor in bringing about this great victory, and special mention was made of the fact that the women of the "Nursing Settlement" on Henry Street had been largely influential in rousing the women of upper New York to a knowledge of the terrible conditions that existed in the slum districts under Tammany rule.

This circumstance is of interest to the profession at large, for the reason that nurses, for the first time, were given recognition as political reformers, a place that, in the future, they would fill with great honor.

JANUARY 1902

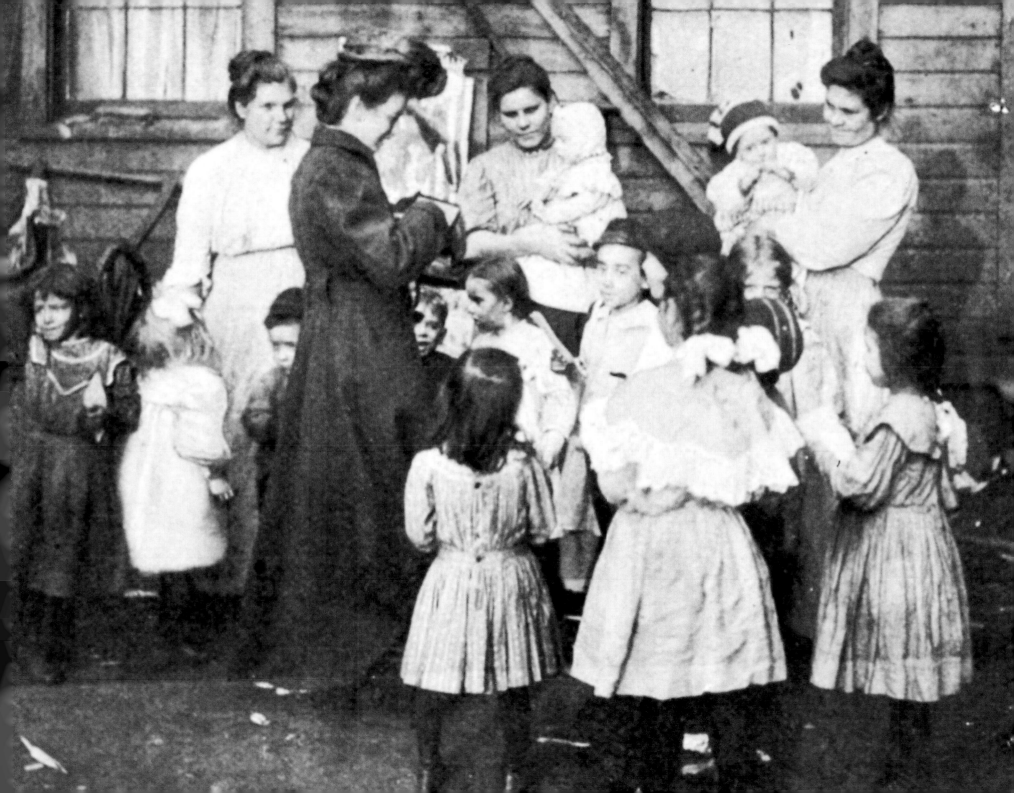

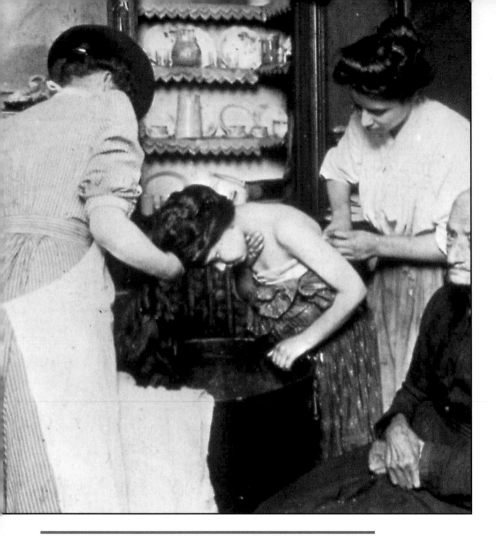

Boston visiting nurse assisting a mother with her sick daughter.

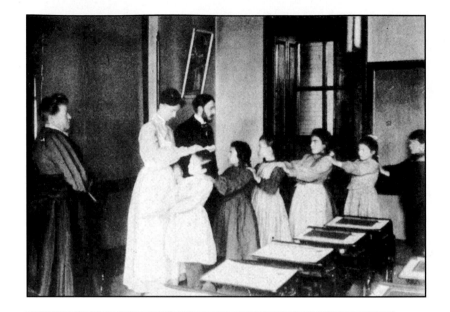

The placement of nurses in schools began in New York City in 1902 at the urging of Lillian Wald, who offered to supply a Henry Street nurse for one month without cost to prove her belief in their worth.

Tuberculosis patient taking fresh air treatment on roof.

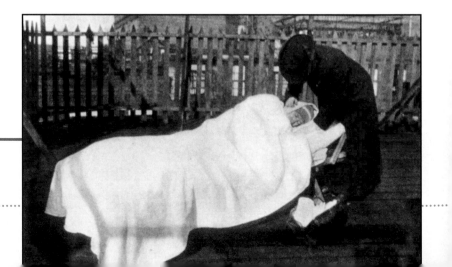

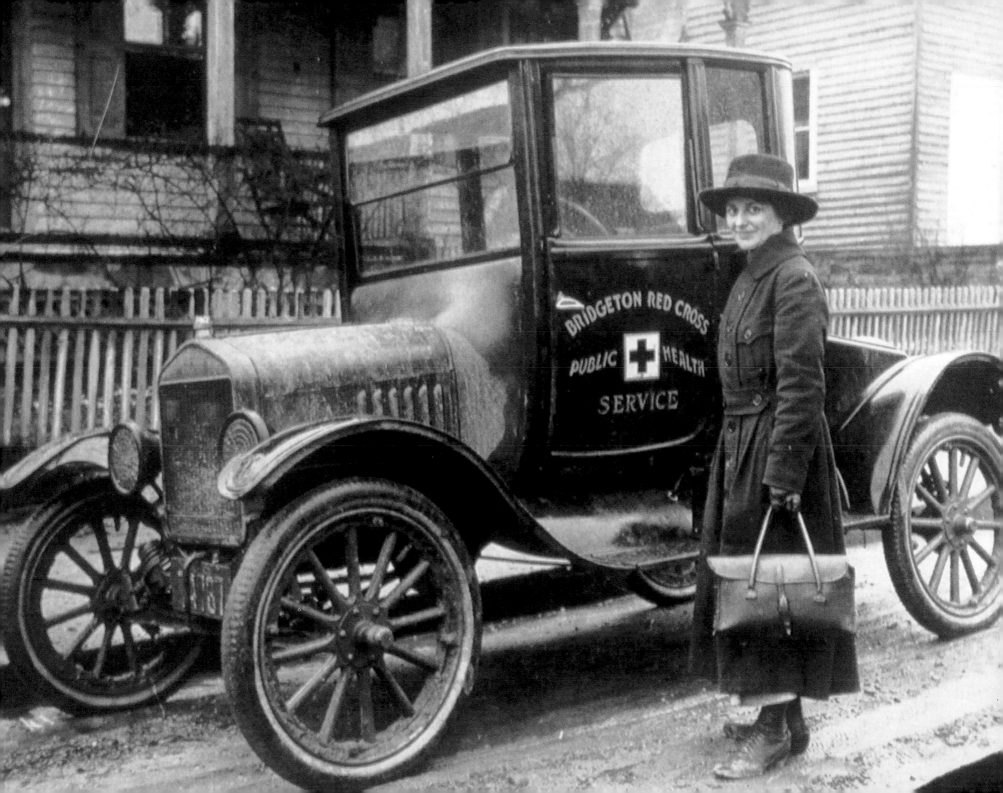

Candy Factories Healthful

A London physician has lately expressed the opinion that both candy and sealing-wax factories are very healthful places in which to work. The candy girls, he says, are allowed to eat as much sugar as they like, with an excellent effect upon their health. Experience shows that the sugar eater is proof against consumption, and it is impossible for her to become a drunkard. The resin dust in the sealing-wax factories makes the air in them very stimulating, similar to that of a pine forest. It is true that the workers in these factories inevitably absorb with the dust particles of vermilion coloring, which is a virulent poison; but, according to the optimistic writer, even this has a good effect upon anemics.

OCTOBER 1907

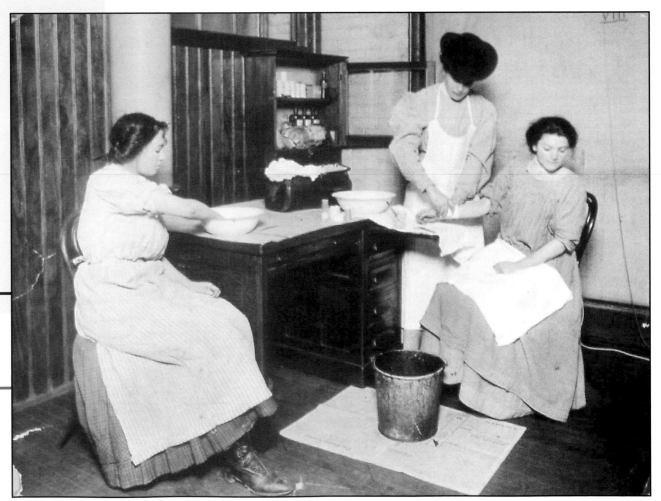

First Aid Room in a 1909 chocolate factory.

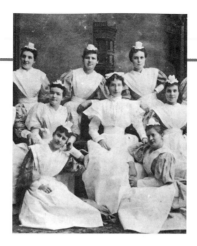

Commentary

Nettie Birnbach

Registration

The nurse registration movement, begun in 1893, is a significant milestone in the history of American caregiving. Representing the earliest unified effort to achieve licensure for qualified practitioners, the registration movement reflected concern for and commitment to the public welfare and status of the individual nurse.

During the 1890s, hospital authorities gradually recognized the advantages to be gained from retaining a ready supply of inexpensive labor, and, as new hospitals and sanitariums emerged, training schools were incorporated into many of those facilities. Between 1890 and 1900, approximately four hundred training schools for nurses were established. The absence of uniformity in content and length of program resulted in nurses with markedly differing abilities. Unfortunately, the public lacked the knowledge to distinguish between nurses who were well prepared and those who were not. Graduates of the earliest training programs, who ultimately assumed leadership positions as superintendents of the more reputable schools, became increasingly alarmed by the flagrant disregard for standards demonstrated by ambitious entrepreneurs who exploited student nurses for financial gain. These factors, plus the unchecked proliferation of all kinds of training schools, including correspondence schools, provoked the need for legal controls and provided the impetus for reform.

Between 1890 and 1902, the gathering momentum for registration led to the formation of state associations that were to implement the strategies for achieving legal regulation. The justification for state promotion of registration laws was in keeping with the states' rights provision of the U.S. Constitution.

In 1901, New York, Virginia, Illinois, and New Jersey, respectively, were the first state associations to organize. In 1903, North Carolina was the first state to enact a registration law. New Jersey, New York, and Virginia followed that same year. By 1909, thirty-three state associations were in existence—twenty-four having attained nursing legislation. In addition, thirty-three practice acts were passed by 1912, forty by 1915, and forty-five by 1917. Twenty years after enactment of the first laws, legislation regulating nursing was operative in forty-eight states, Hawaii, and the District of Columbia. "Registered nurse" was the title incorporated into most of the laws, and almost all provided for the establishment of state boards of examiners.

During the struggle for registration, opposition was encountered from the proprietors of disreputable training schools. The public press was divided, as were public officials, legislators, and the medical community. Among nurses, anti-registration positions were held by those who failed to meet the criteria in the laws and perceived their careers to be in jeopardy. The all-nurse composition of many of the state boards of examiners also elicited criticism. Additionally, problems were encountered by nurses administering the laws, graduate nurses who were slow to apply for registration, training schools that were indifferent to provisions in the legislation, and state-to-state variations in the laws.

Arguably, the most glaring deficiency was the permissive nature of the early practice acts. These acts neither defined nor effectively limited the practice of nursing, and although all the laws included provisions for licensure as a registered nurse, none prohibited the untrained from practicing as nurses. Overall, however, the establishment of practice acts was highly productive. The early laws upgraded nursing school entry requirements, lengthened the program of study, and raised the standards of nursing education in this country. Gradually, repeated amendments and revisions to the laws strengthened their effectiveness. Still, the failure of any state to enact a compulsory licensure law remained problematic.

Throughout the 1930s, organized nursing made numerous attempts to alter the existing permissive statutes. The first mandatory licensure law enacted in New York in 1938 did not take effect until 1949. By the 1970s, a majority of states had enacted compulsory legislation, but many of the laws were

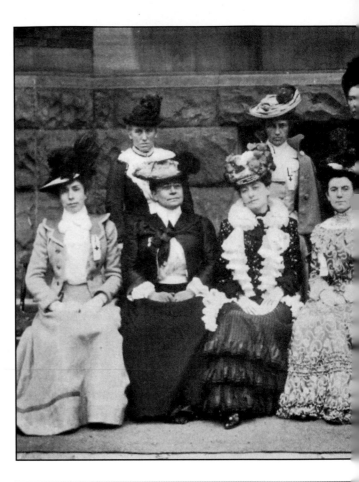

FOREIGN DELEGATES AND OFFICERS, International Congress of Nurses, Buffalo, September 18–21, 1901. Front row (left to right): Miss McGahey, Sydney, Australia; Miss Stewart, London; Mrs. Bedford-Fenwick, London; Miss McIsaac, Chicago; Miss Keating, Buffalo; Miss Damer, Buffalo; Miss Banfield, Philadelphia; Miss Sniveley, Toronto. Back row (left to right): Miss Wood, London; Miss Arkle, Australia; Miss Hughes, England; Miss Mollett, England; Miss Cartwright, London; Miss Waind, England.

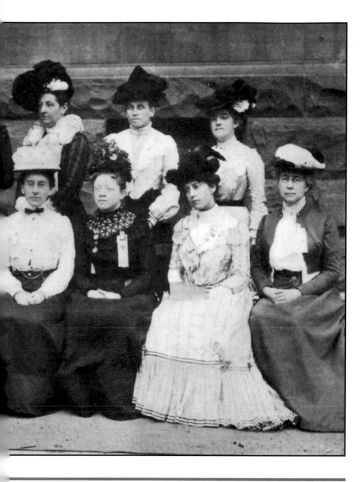

From the very beginning, American nursing has had international connections and, in fact, the impetus for American nurses organizing came from Ethel Bedford-Fenwick, founder of the British Nurses Association.

ambiguous and subject to various interpretations. In 1972, the landmark revision of the New York State Nurse Practice Act became law, and was the first legislation to define nursing practice and recognize nursing's independent role and diagnostic function. Widely adopted by other state nurses' associations, the definition of nursing in the 1972 law was incorporated into ANA's Social Policy Statement. In several states, the recent enactment of laws generating a second license for advanced practice has created enormous controversy. Over time, opposition to nursing's advancement persisted. The recurring threat of institutional licensure, for example, arose from those who believe that individual licensure is no longer justifiable and that employing institutions should be responsible for credentialing their personnel.

With respect to the early state boards of examiners, limitations to their effectiveness became apparent. The absence of guidelines for validating competency compromised the tests. Nurses preparing the examinations were often inexperienced in test question construction and, with each state administering its own examination, reliability varied from state-to-state. These inconsistencies deterred interstate mobility for nurses.

By 1928, nursing leaders began discussing the feasibility of forming a national board of examiners whose members would create a standard qualifying examination acceptable to all state boards. The Council of State Boards in Nursing was launched as a result of those discussions.

The successful development of a national examination, the State Board Test Pool Exam (SBTPE), was largely the work of R. Louise McManus of Teachers College, Columbia University. Between 1944 and 1950, the SBTPE became the approved test for all states. An early problem involving differences in acceptable passing scores among states was resolved when a uniform passing grade was adopted. In 1982, a newly designed examination, the N-CLEX, was implemented. Currently, the test is computerized to ease student access.

In 1979, the status of the Council of State Boards changed. At that time, the Council was subsidized by the ANA, which raised the issue of potential conflict of interest. The outcome of these problems was the founding of an independent organization, the National Council of State Boards of Nursing, Inc. (NCSBN). Recently, the NCSBN adopted a resolution endorsing "a mutual recognition model of nursing regulation," which, in effect, creates a multistate system of licensure. Once again, the subject of credentialing for nurses is stirring controversy within the profession. And, once more, state associations are taking action to protect their practice acts. For the moment, the RN credential remains intact.

COMMENT

The code of ethics, which had been presented at a previous meeting and laid upon the table, was taken up and discussed. In this connection was read a paper written by Miss Lavinia L. Dock, secretary of the International Council of Nurses, on "Ethics in Nursing." This was both bright and trite. Recess was then taken, when refreshments were served and an opportunity was given the members to discuss the proposed code informally.

FEBRUARY 1901

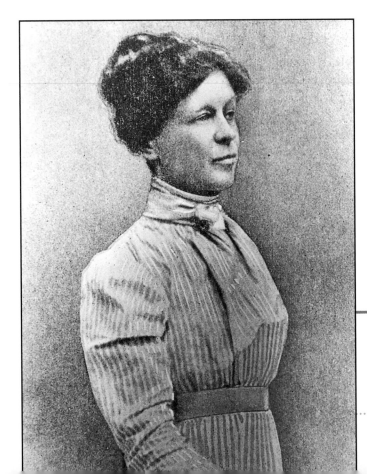

Lavinia Lloyd Dock

Miss Dock was far ahead of her time in recognizing the importance of organized effort to create or influence public opinion. She was present at the meeting in Chicago, in 1893, at which the first of our national associations—the American Society of Superintendents of Training Schools for Nurses—was conceived, and she became its first secretary. She was one of the far-seeing supporters of two of the early projects of that organization: the launching of the Associated Alumnae (later the American Nurses Association) and the securing of an entree for nursing at Teachers College, Columbia University. She purchased stock in the embryonic American Journal of Nursing Company and subsequently served for more than twenty years as editor of the magazine's Foreign Department (1900–1923). . . . Deeply compassionate, intellectually forthright and far-seeing, happily and often amusingly unconventional, she became mildly a militant suffragist.

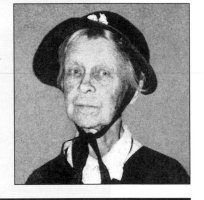

By 1900, Lavinia Dock was already a recognized nursing leader.

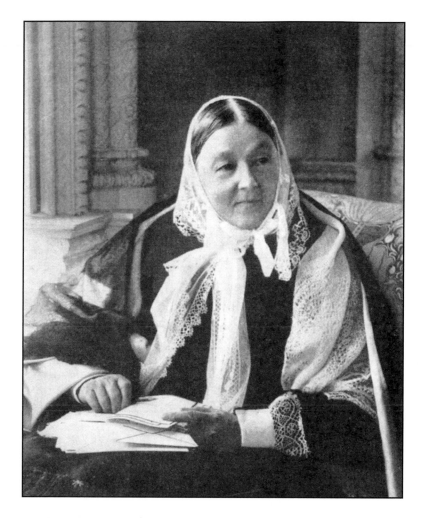

Miss Nightingale in later life, from a photograph that she particularly liked. This portrait hangs in the Anna C. Maxwell Hall at Columbia-Presbyterian Medical Center in New York City. It was secured through the courtesy of the *Nursing Mirror* of London, by Eleanor Creighton of England, an aunt of Mrs. Hugh Auchincloss. This picture was presented to the nursing school's Florence Nightingale Collection in May 1939, by the late Dr. Hugh Auchincloss, who made many gifts to the collection.

COMMENT

The Death of Florence Nightingale

Florence Nightingale passed from this visible world on August 13, having completed her ninetieth year. Probably the image of her which we all carry in our hearts is that of the youthful, gracious presence which the soldiers loved and blessed, and which all men honored—yet a full half century has passed since her work in the Crimea. . . .

In thinking of her work and influence, we must avoid the mistake of picturing her appearance at that dark time, fifty years ago, as that of a meteor, suddenly shining in the night and then disappearing. Miss Nightingale accomplished her great mission in life, not by chance or accident, nor was her influence due wholly to her wonderful natural gifts and graces. Without the most careful training and preparation, even her angelic goodness and magnetic influence might have been of but little lasting benefit.

The more we study her life and her writings, the more we must be amazed at the reach of her vision, for she was the first thinker and writer of her times on hygiene, on hospital and training-school administration, on private and hospital nursing methods, and on the care of the sick poor in their own homes. Although her presentation of these subjects is clear and convincing, humanitarians have been slow in learning the lesson, and are just beginning to catch up with her in their comprehension of these problems.

SEPTEMBER, 1910

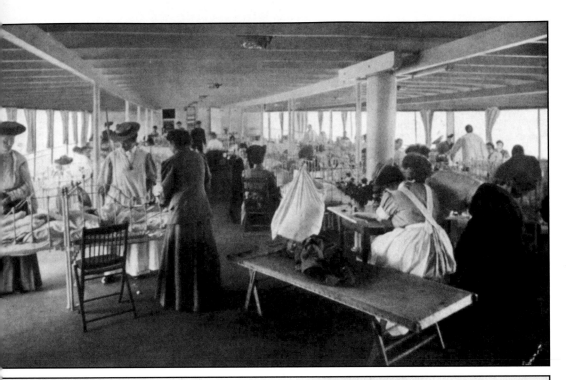

The Boston Floating Hospital, and later the New York Floating Hospital, were designed to provide education in maternal and child care to graduate nurses and to give indigent mothers and children a "pleasant day on the water." Meals, health examinations, and patient education were provided in a day-long sail.

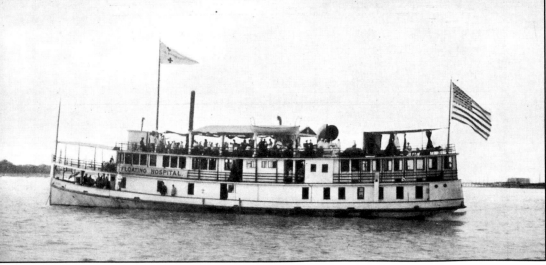

The Boston Floating Hospital, 1905.

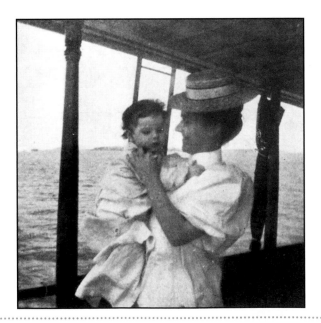

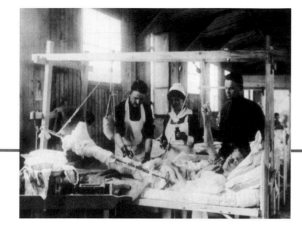

The Great War and Its Aftermath

1914–1929

In April, 1917, the United States entered into World War I, a war unlike any it had ever known. Three and a half million men joined the U.S. Army, and two million of them were sent to France to fight. Within a month, M. Adelaide Nutting called a meeting of nursing leaders and organized a National Emergency Committee on Nursing. In August, this group became attached to the General Medical Board of the U.S. Council of National Defense, and functioned as the national center responsible for meeting military and civilian demands for nursing services. It also worked closely with the Red Cross Nursing Service that served as the military reserve, enrolling and supplying nurses to expand the Army and Navy Nurse Corps.

In order to train large numbers of skilled nurses to fill the needs brought on by the war, the Committee on Nursing instituted the Army School of Nursing and the Vassar Training Camp, in addition to the Student Nurse Reserve. The Army School of Nursing was developed as a training program for nurses that featured academics and direct training in army hospitals. The Vassar Camp, which included academic preparation on college grounds and training in cooperating hospital schools of nursing, paved the way for incorporating nursing education into institutions of higher learning. During this time, the General Medical Board also appealed to leading nursing schools around the country to expand enrollments.

As the war waged on and the fighting in France and Belgium grew more vicious, Army and Navy nurses stationed overseas cared for soldiers with more devastating wounds than they could ever have imagined—from bullets, shrapnel, shells, chlorine, and mustard gas. The number of casualties grew and the Army Nurse Corps swelled to 21,000; the Navy, to almost 1,500.

Meanwhile, in September 1918, the great influenza epidemic broke out and would ultimately take more lives than the war had. In the United States alone, more than a half million people died. Worldwide, the number was estimated at 25 million. Again, nurses were called upon to care for the multitude.

In the United States, the influenza epidemic was at its peak by the time news of the armistice was received in November 1918.

Immediately after the war, health care in the United States was disorganized and nurses were in short supply. Many graduate and student nurses had themselves fallen victim to the disease. Hospitals were still recovering from the war and the influenza outbreak and were trying to rebuild. To meet these needs and to ensure a low-cost ready supply of caregivers, hospital training schools began forming at an alarming rate. Soon there were a high number of students enrolled in the schools. With only a small percentage of hospital budgets being allocated for the schools, however, the quality of instruction and training materials was low, and many students were graduating with an inadequate education. Critics at the time argued that nursing education could not advance until schools were removed from hospitals and assumed control over their own finances.

In 1919, a Committee for the Study of Nursing Education, supported by the Rockefeller Foundation, was initially set up to examine public health nursing education, and was then broadened to study nursing education in general. The end product was the Goldmark Report, released in 1923, which was quoted extensively throughout the century for its criticism of the way hospital training schools were being run, too often sacrificing the needs of students to the demands of service.

In 1926, the Committee on the Grading of Nursing Schools was organized and financed with a $93,000 grant from Frances Payne Bolton, who sat on the committee and had endowed the new school of nursing at Western Reserve University in Cleveland, Ohio in 1924. The group focused on the supply of and demand for nurses; a job analysis of what nursing entailed and how students should be prepared; and an evaluation of the quality of existing schools of nursing. *Nurses, Patients, and Pocketbooks*, published in 1928, indicated that there was an oversupply of nurses who were inadequately and unevenly trained, and significantly underpaid. It was clear that nurses needed to take control over the direction of their profession.

Noble Crusader

Lillian Wald (1867–1940), often compared to Florence Nightingale, was a person "with the creative imagination we call genius," statesmanship, and access to influence and money to fund the many programs and institutions she conceived. Among them were the Henry Street Settlement and the New York Visiting Nurse Service; public health nursing and the National Organization of Public Health Nursing (NOPHN); school nursing; the Metropolitan Life Insurance Company Nursing Service; the Children's Bureau; the Town and Country Nursing Service of the American Red Cross; the introduction of social services into municipal hospitals and many more civic, political, and health achievements.

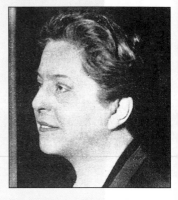

LILLIAN D. WALD, RN

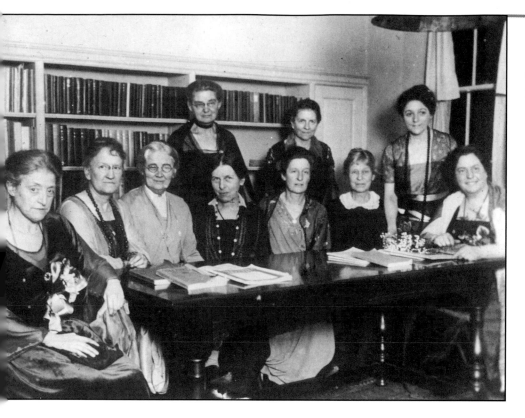

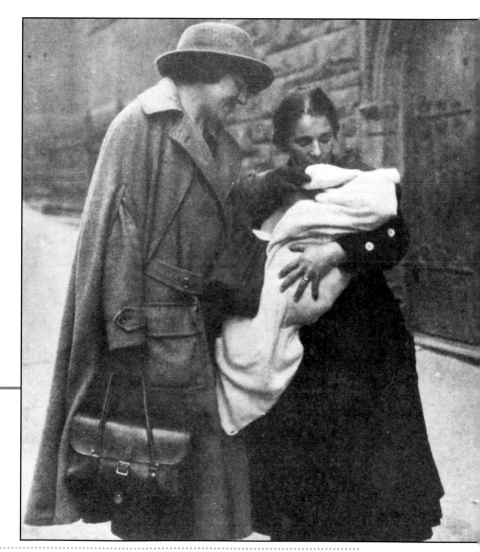

Notable women who have contributed to the success of Henry Street (left to right): Annie W. Goodrich, Jane E. Hitchcock, Georgiana B. Judson, M. Adelaide Nutting, Henrietta Van Cleft, Rebecca Shatz, Mary Magoun Brown, Lavinia L. Dock, Elizabeth A. Frank, Lillian D. Wald.

A Henry Street visiting nurse meets a proud mother.

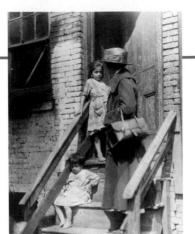

Commentary

Virginia Ohlson and Jean Wood

Public Health and Community Health Nursing

Initially, public health nursing was service directed to the sick poor in their homes and was funded by voluntary and philanthropic organizations and individuals. The mission of public health nursing practice emphasized health promotion and disease prevention rather than the curative and palliative care provided by the institutions of the day. Attending to the family environment, teaching the care of the sick to patients and family members, and teaching good hygiene practices to all family members were important characteristics of the nurses' practice. As local and state government began to assume responsibility for the health and welfare of its citizens, public health nursing became a part of health department programs.

With the evolution of public health nursing practice, service was directed to a wide spectrum of people defined by geographic boundaries (city, county, district, parish), special populations (mothers and infants, school-age children, working adults), or a specific health problem of a population group (communicable disease, tuberculosis, venereal disease). In all situations, the public health team practiced with a high degree of autonomy, in collaboration with the community. Significant to the organization of the service was the involvement of individuals interested in bettering the health of others. Lillian Wald was the first person to use the term "public health nurse," and it was her goal to make it known to the public that the public health nurse was their nurse.

Professionalization of public health nursing was a counterpart to the development of practice. Lillian Wald, together with other nursing leaders of the day, formed the National Organization for Public Health Nursing (NOPHN) and she became its first president This organization had two purposes: to standardize public health nursing practice and to further the relationships among all people interested in the public's health. The leadership of this organization achieved quality and standardization for public health nursing practice through accreditation of programs and certification of prac-

THE
PUBLIC HEALTH NURSE

She Answers Humanity's Call
Your Red Cross Membership
makes her work possible.

In 1917, a group of government investigators made a series of studies in rural communities of conditions affecting maternal and child welfare. They found a great need for educational health work and a need for the care of the sick and for the correction of defects. They were often asked to make recommendations, and among other things their outstanding reply was, "Get a public health nurse."

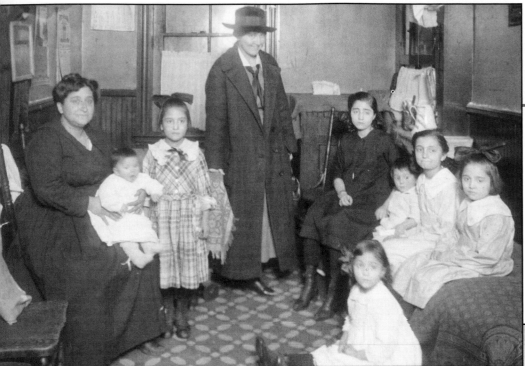

A Boston visiting nurse attending to a large family on North Margin Street, circa 1920.

Visiting nurses routing reports in office at Boston's South end.

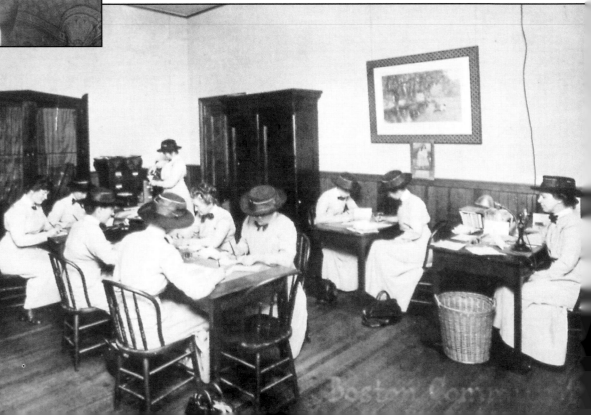

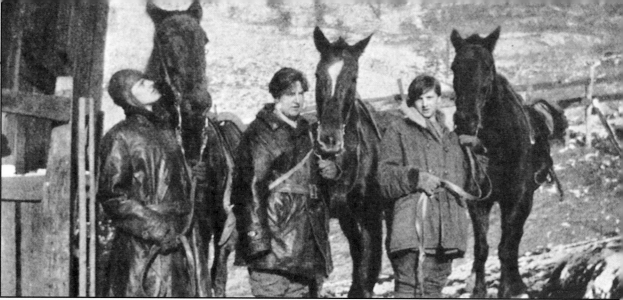

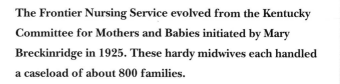
The Frontier Nursing Service evolved from the Kentucky Committee for Mothers and Babies initiated by Mary Breckinridge in 1925. These hardy midwives each handled a caseload of about 800 families.

titioners. Public health nursing leaders were at the forefront of the effort to place the education of nurses within colleges and universities. The first baccalaureate degrees offered in nursing were the bachelor of science in public health nursing (BSPHN) and the bachelor of science in nursing education (BSNE). Over time, professional nursing recognized that preparation for specialty practice was more appropriate for graduate study, and that baccalaureate education was basic to the practice of all nursing.

In the 1980s, the American Nurses Association realigned its membership structure and the title community health nursing was given to the public health nursing membership unit. This change paved the way for a single grouping of all members employed outside of hospital settings regardless of their educational preparation, philosophy or mission of practice, or unit of service (individual, family, or community). But the public health nursing specialist has not been willing to give up the philosophy and theory of public health. Hence, the term "public health/community health nursing."

In the twentieth century, public health/community health nursing took root. In the twenty-first century, its evolution will be determined by the practitioners' ability to remain focused on health promotion and disease prevention for the good of the public's health. Practitioners will be required to exert leadership within the communities in which they work to incorporate within society not only the value of fixing health problems, but also of preventing their occurrence.

Letters

Dear Editor:

The case of which I wish to tell you was at Glyndon, Minnesota, several miles out of town, where the prairie meets the horizon in every direction. The attending physician met me with his auto in Fargo, and while going to the home the doctor was preparing me for what I was going to get into, but to the worst things he would mention, I always said, "I don't mind."

On opening the door, I got the foul odor of diphtheria, and I saw two children lying on the floor on a bed of old, soiled quilts and coats, with swollen throats and staring eyes and the grey diphtheria membrane extending from their noses. On entering another room, we found the warm dead body of little Edith with golden curls. The room was in a terribly disordered condition. And while all this was taking place, the mother of the three children was in the Rochester, Minnesota, Hospital with very badly swollen limbs, in a nervous condition entirely uncontrollable.

August 1916

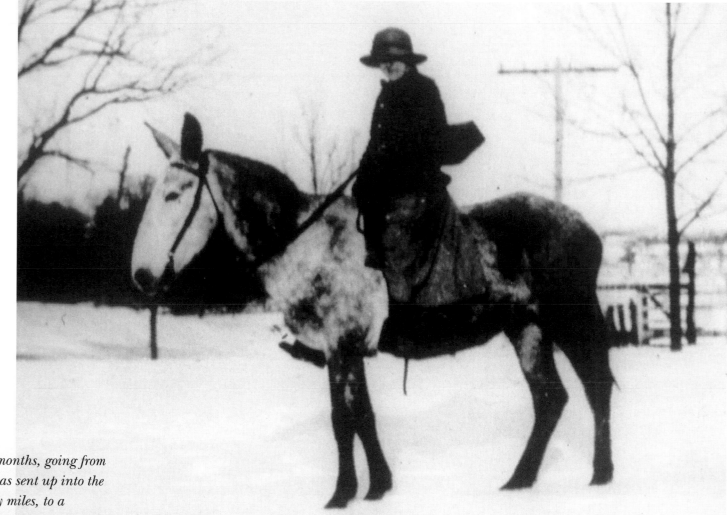

"After three or four months, going from one case to another, I was sent up into the mountains, about thirty miles, to a typhoid fever case. My medicine for this case was a package of epsom salt."

BILLINGS, MONTANA, 1914

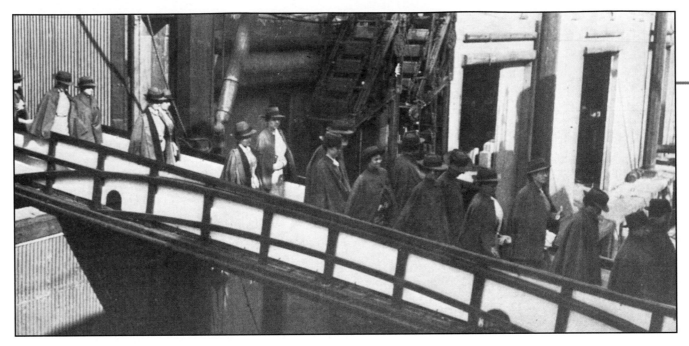

Leaving for the war zone.

The Nurse on the Docks

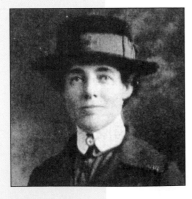

A mental picture of Florence Johnson's erect and gallant figure in uniform, and her friendly words of cheer and admonition have been cherished through the years by thousands of veterans of World War I who have had pride in recalling that "She saw our unit off!" Thus was begun a service which gave her the sobriquet "the nurse on the docks" and an honored and unique place in the history of nursing.

Nurse of the #326th Field Hospital bathing the eyes of gassed patients from the 82nd and 89th Divisions north of Royaumeix, France in 1919. The gassed patients present one of the saddest sights to be seen, with their eyes swollen and discharging, the body covered with blisters, with the accompanying pain, and with apparent discomfort in the respiratory tract which, having a moist mucous surface, is affected seriously. These patients expectorate quantities of blood and nearly all are unable to speak above a whisper. In a single day seven hundred of these patients were admitted.

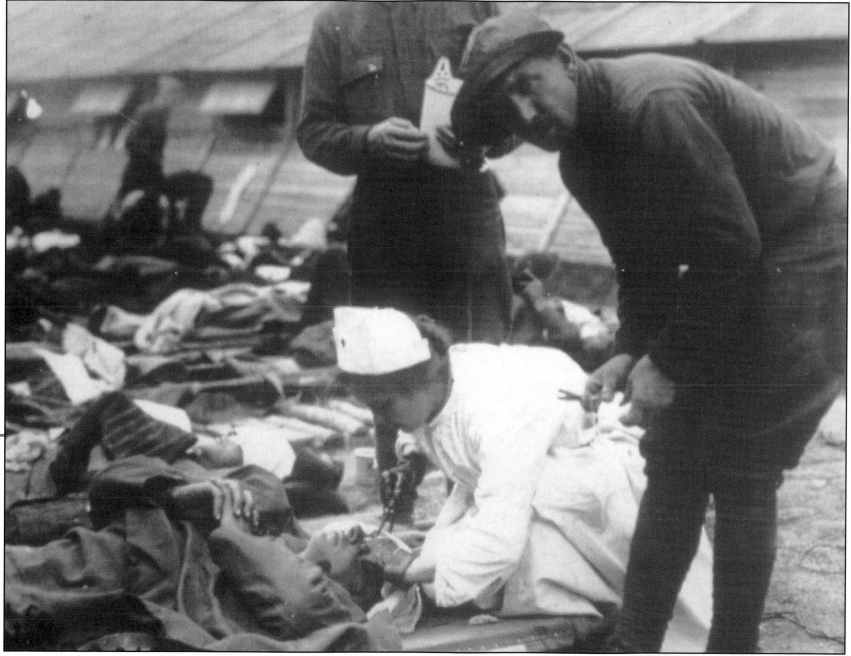

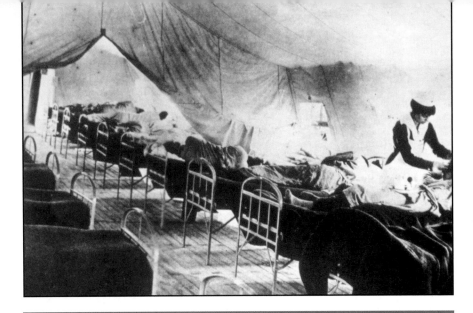

Interior of ward # 3, at American Red Cross Hospital. Auteuil, Paris, France.

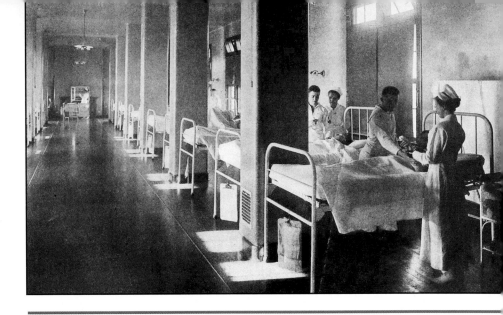

A ward in the Naval Hospital, Puget Sound.

Heroic Nurse

Edith Cavell, a 49-year-old British nurse, was executed by the Germans in 1915 for harboring Allied soldiers in occupied Belgium—not, as many assume, for spying. She held the position of matron in a Belgian hospital at the time the war broke out.

The penalty which Miss Cavell paid by her death is the same, we suppose, as would have been meted out to a man under similar conditions and we may all glory in the fact that she met her death with the same courage and fortitude that the world expects from its great soldiers.

NOVEMBER 1915

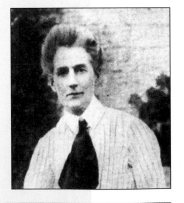

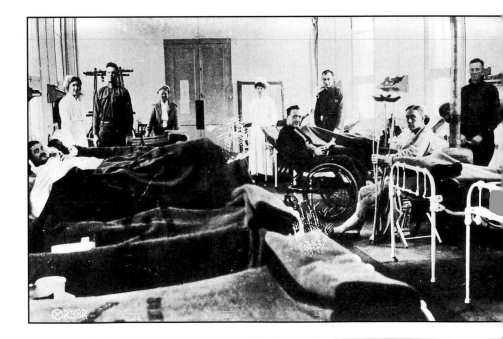

Our own nurses care for our own men, over there.

Letter from France

"No lights were allowed after 7 p.m. but we could have a small candle to look after the wounded if the windows were closely screened. We heard the shells whistling through the air and waited for the house to shake after the explosion. Houses near us caught fire, others collapsed. We were too busy to mind in the daytime but at night it was rather weird. I often looked out of the window and watched those terrific fireworks which, if they had not brought death and destruction in their wake, would have been impressive with their magnificence.

The last week of the bombardment, when the town itself was being shelled, the 19 St. John nurses were asked by the British consulate if they would like to leave, as a boat was ready to take them to England, and although we were all separated and none knew what the others had decided, no one took advantage of the offer, nor did I hear of any nurses leaving the town. They all stayed in their hospitals."

June 1915

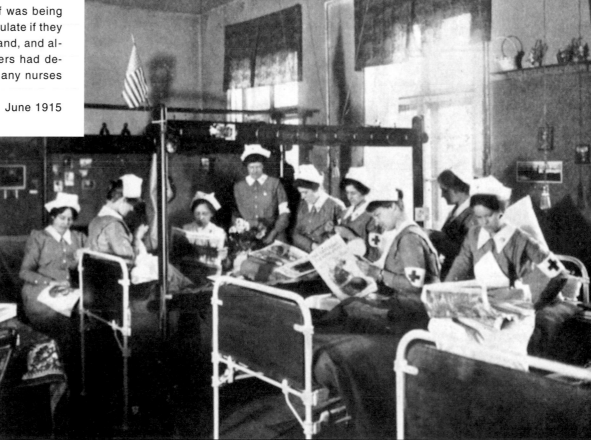

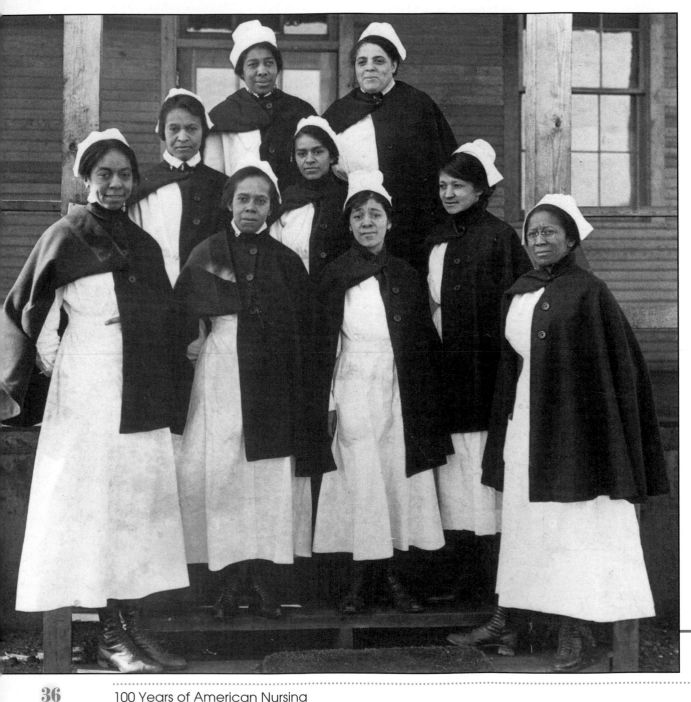

"Despite their honorable service in the Spanish-American War in 1898, there were no black nurses among the members of the Army Nurse Corps when it was formally established in 1901. And, despite the efforts of NACGN and others, those black nurses who had volunteered their services during World War I were not accepted by the Army Nurse Corps until after the Armistice had been signed in 1918 and only 18 were accepted at that time. Their acceptance was, no doubt, due to the great need for nurses during the influenza pandemic."

M. ELIZABETH CARNEGIE

Black nurses at Camp Sherman in Chillicothe, Ohio in 1918.

The Vassar Training Camp of 1918 was an intensive three-month experimental program designed to interest college graduates in nursing. A total of 439 women enrolled for the summer course on the Vassar campus, which provided all the preparatory courses and would be followed by two years of clinical experience at one of the 33 cooperating hospital schools of nursing. Of the 439, 418 completed the Vassar course and 399 entered the affiliated nursing schools. As a result of this success, similar courses were set up at Western Reserve, the University of Cincinnati, the University of Iowa, the University of Colorado, and the University of California.

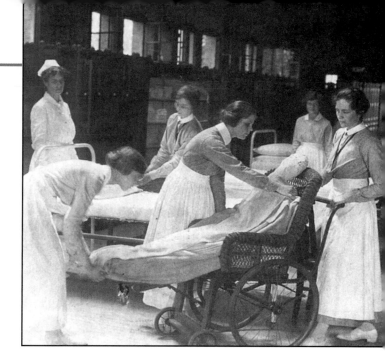

Students learning nursing fundamentals at the Vassar College program.

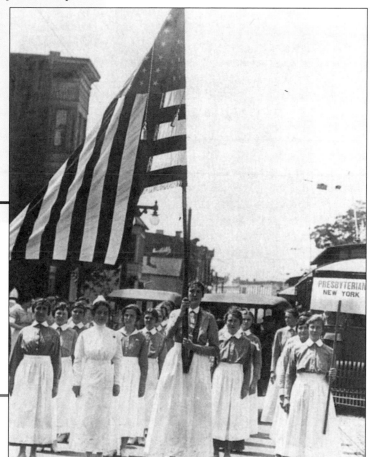

Student nurses in the experimental program at Vassar College parade for the public.

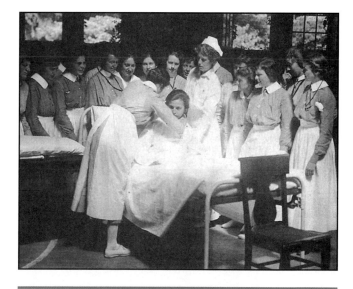

These Vassar students would go on to complete their nurses' training at cooperating hospital schools.

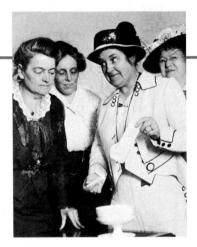

Commentary

Robert Piemonte

Nursing Organizations

A major push toward organization took place in the 1920s, although the forming of alliances began earlier. Nurses in North America came together in a general meeting for the first time at the International Congress of Charities, Correction, and Philanthropy at the Chicago World's Fair on June 15–17, 1893. Ethel Bedford-Fenwick, founder of the British Nurses Association, arranged a subsection in nursing at the convention, which was chaired by Isabel Hampton (later Robb). Hampton was assisted by M. Adelaide Nutting and Lavinia L. Dock in planning a program that focused on control of nurse training schools, the registration of nurses, and the formation of a national organization.

Nurses at the meeting spoke on many issues of concern to the fledgling profession. For example, Edith A. Draper discussed the need for an American Nurses Association, Isabel McIsaac lectured on the benefits of alumnae associations, and Isabel Hampton articulated a need for the establishment of both an organization of alumnae associations and a nursing school superintendents' society before the establishment of a national association of nurses.

The 18 superintendents of training schools present at the conference met before the congress ended to discuss forming a society. On June 16, 1893, the superintendents adopted resolutions to establish the American Society of Superintendents of Training Schools for Nurses. Goals of the society were to promote fellowship among nurses, establish and maintain a

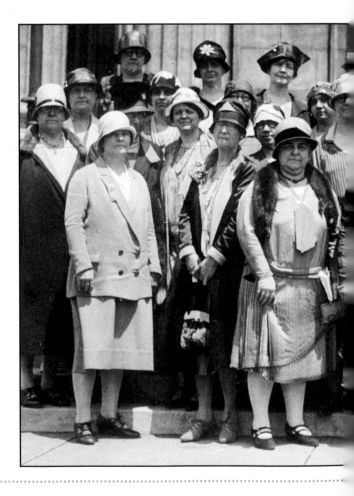

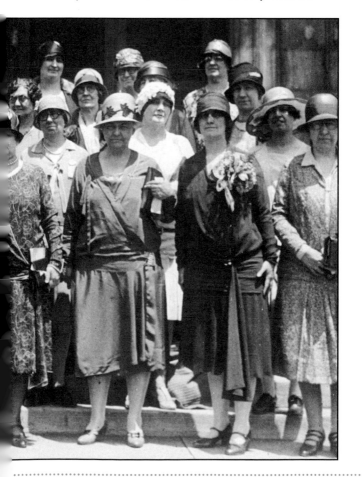

Early arrivals for the 1928 ANA Advisory Council.

universal standard of training, and further the best interests of the profession. The society's first convention was held in New York City on January 10, 1894. At this time, a constitution and bylaws were approved, and Linda Richards was elected president.

During the early years, the society worked diligently to stimulate interest in forming a national association of trained nurses. At the second annual convention, Sophia F. Palmer presented a paper on school alumnae associations. Palmer believed that the power of the profession depended on its ability to maintain the cooperation of individual nurses who could influence public opinion.

At the third convention, Lavinia L. Dock spoke on establishing and organizing a national association. Following her presentation, a Committee for the Organization of a National Association for Nurses was appointed and charged with drafting a constitution. The committee met in September, 1896, in New York City, and determined that the organization be named the Associated Alumnae of the United States and Canada. A constitution and bylaws were adopted at the organization's first meeting, which was held February 11–12, 1897, in Baltimore, during the society's fourth annual convention. The objectives identified by the organization were to establish and maintain a code of ethics; to elevate the standards of nursing education; and to promote the usefulness, honor, and financial interests of the nursing profession. Isabel Hampton Robb was elected the first president and served until September, 1901.

In 1900, the Nurses' Associated Alumnae affiliated with the American Society of Superintendents of Training Schools for Nurses so that they might apply for membership in the National Council of Women. The collaboration, entitled the American Federation of Nurses, was accepted for membership in 1901. In 1904, the American Federation of Nurses, the National Council of Nurses in England, and the German Nurses Association were invited to join the International Council of Nurses.

It is important to note that these nursing alliances were composed of white women only. Patterns of discrimination were so strong that African American nurses felt the need to establish their own organization, and in 1908, the National Association of Colored Graduate Nurses was formed. For several decades, the struggle for equal treatment continued.

As nursing grew, so did the profession's special interests. The dawn of the twentieth century brought an increase in the work of community health nurses in cities and rural communities. Consequently, visiting nurse societies were established to meet public health needs. On June 7, 1912, the National Organization for Public Health Nursing was established, and Lillian Wald was elected its first president.

By 1912, the names of some of these organizations had changed to reflect an expanding vision. The Associated Alumnae became the American Nurses Association, and the American Society of Superintendents of Training Schools for Nurses became the National League of Nursing Education.

A special conference on nursing programs within colleges and universities was held at Teachers College, Columbia University, in January 1933. The conference resulted in the founding of the Association of Collegiate Schools of Nursing. At the first annual meeting, held in 1934 at Yale University, 19 schools qualified for membership. Among concerns discussed were length of nursing courses and clinical experience. Annie Goodrich and Isabel Stewart were among the most active representatives of member schools.

By 1945, seven national nursing organizations had been established: the National League of Nursing Education (1893), the American Nurses Association (1897), the National Association of Colored Graduate Nurses (1908), the National Organization for Public Health Nursing (1912), the American Association of Nurse Anesthetists (1931), the Association of Collegiate Schools of Nursing (1933), and the American Association of Industrial Nurses (1942).

In 1946, Raymond Rich Associates was commissioned to study the structural principles essential for the effective operation of the existing nursing organizations. Acting on the study results, which suggested consolidation, the House of Delegates at the 1952 American Nurses Association Convention approved plans for a restructuring into two major organizations—the American Nurses Association (ANA) and the National League for Nursing (NLN). As the plan took shape, the National Association of Colored Graduate Nurses, the National Organization for Public Health Nursing, and the Association of Collegiate Schools of Nursing dissolved, their functions being subsumed within the ANA and NLN.

In spite of efforts to streamline, as nursing became more complex, and as specialty practice evolved, new groups organized around practice issues. There are currently more than 30 specialty nursing organizations. Moreover, Sigma Theta Tau International, the professional honor society of nursing founded in 1922, now has more than 400 chapters in colleges and universities offering baccalaureate and higher degree programs.

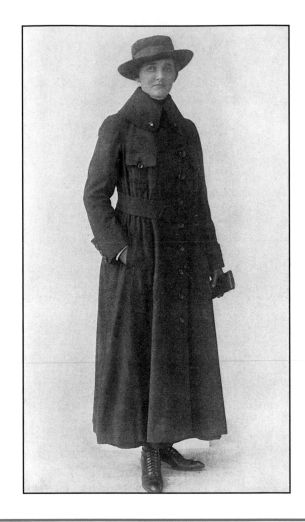

"After ten years of service, my Red Cross cape is now on its way back to you. . . . It has kept me warm and dry during many days of hard labor in the field. In South Texas I used to hang it on the door of the car, red side out, and the mothers watched for that signal to bring their children to the health center, or to meet me at the roadside on my return. . . . I hope that I have always worn it worthily. . . ."

AUGUST 1929

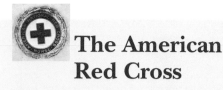

The American Red Cross

The American Red Cross (ARC) was created by Congressional charter in 1905 to provide aid and relief service during war as well as during national emergencies in peacetime. In 1909, the nursing service was organized with Jane Delano as the first chairman. During World War I, the ARC served as the official reserve, charged with recruiting, equipping, and assigning nurses for the 49 base hospitals operated by the Army and eight Navy base hospitals, as well as their own Red Cross hospitals. In 1918, the ARC worked with the American Nurses Association on a national nursing survey. There were 98,162 graduate nurses in the United States.

In 1918, the Red Cross Town and Country Nursing Service became the Bureau of Public Health Nursing Service and was charged with improving sanitary conditions in army camps where the influenza epidemic of 1918 was causing chaos. Following the war, ARC nurses cared for displaced and ill refugees, war orphans, disabled and sick nurses, and soldiers at home and abroad.

The first national congress in nursing was called by the American Association of Critical Care Nurses (AACN) in San Clemente, California, in January 1973. The meeting was organized for the purpose of seeking mutual support and cooperation among specialty nursing groups and the ANA. The 17 organizations attending the meeting formed a 13-member federation with four auditors. The continuing education unit was adopted as the basis for standardizing continuing education for all nursing organizations. Since its inception, the National Federation of Specialty Organizations (NFSNO) has more than doubled its size.

All nursing organizations are invited to come together to discuss mutual concerns through the Nursing Organization Liaison Forum (NOLF), a functional unit of the ANA. Only in this way can nurses speak with one voice. Today, cooperation and flexibility among all nursing organizations are essential if the profession is to advance.

American Red Cross nurses ready to sail.

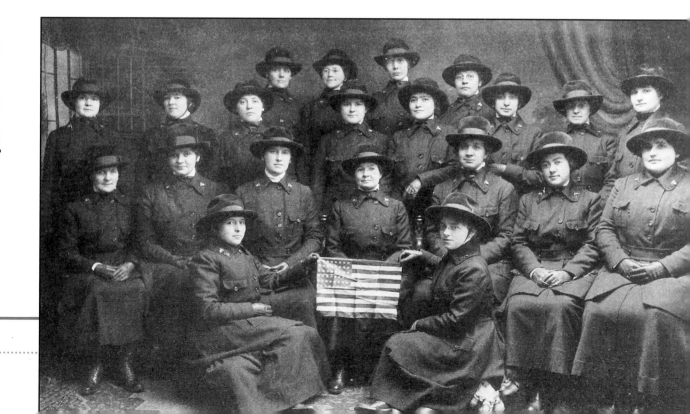

Service Flag of the Department of Nursing bears testimony to the services of American women in the struggle which has just ended. A single blue star represents the 19,877 Red Cross nurses who have been in active duty with the Army and Navy Nurse Corps, and the Red Cross, overseas.

In memory of those nurses who have "gone west," 198 gold stars shine on this service flag. The first to appear were for Mrs. Edith B. Ayres and Helen Burnett Wood, both from Chicago, who were killed May 20, 1917, by the explosion of a defective shell on board the S. S. Mongolia while on their way to France with an early unit. One by one during the early days of our participation in the war, these stars began to appear. The influenza epidemic claimed 81 Red Cross nurses in cantonment hospitals in this country alone. The toll was also great overseas. Two sisters, Viola and Ruth Lundholm, of Oakland, California, contracted this disease while on their way to France and were buried together at Madgalen Hill cemetery, Winchester, England, while others slipped away in Scotland, in France, in Belgium. Even in Germany, there is a white cross marking the grave of Jessie Baldwin, of Summerville, Pa., who died in line of duty, February 6, 1919, at Coblenz, Germany. The last goldstar that has been sewn on this service flag is in memory of Jane A. Delano.

OCTOBER, 1919

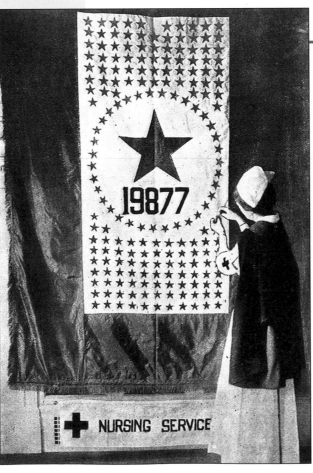

Fastening on the Gold Star for Jane A. Delano.

Head of the Red Cross

Miss Delano's interest in the Red Cross came from her experience in the yellow fever epidemic in Florida, where she served as a volunteer under Clara Barton, then head of the Red Cross. Miss Delano was at the head of the Army Nurse Corps at the time of her appointment as chief of the Red Cross Nursing Service, and held both positions for three years. She was president of the American Nurses' Association from 1909 to 1911.

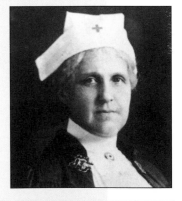

OCTOBER 1919

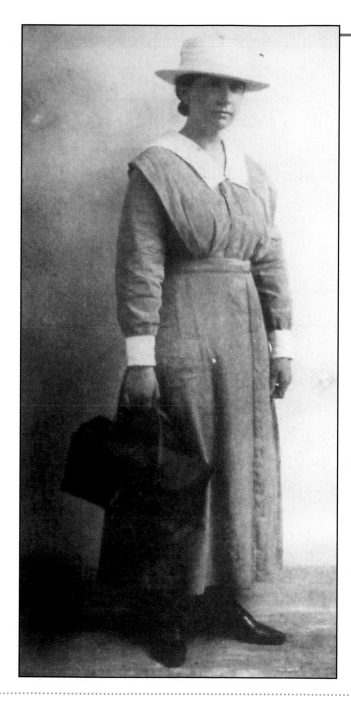

The Red Cross Town and Country nurse is a beloved figure in rural communities scattered from the Atlantic to the Pacific, from Canada to Mexico. Her insignia is the Red Cross pin. To her district she is nurse, mother, sister, teacher and fairy-godmother. In a week she attends the sick, instructs mothers, gives the school children lessons in hygiene, organizes health committees and clubs, brings clean-up and public-welfare campaigns to the country, apparently carrying in her bag a new lease of life for all to whom it opens.

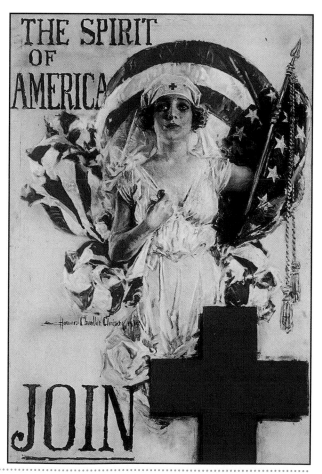

Influenza—1918

On September 21, 1918, the New York City Health Department reported 31 cases of influenza, all in the borough of Brooklyn, with one fatality. This announced the arrival of the devastating Spanish influenza epidemic, which in six short weeks in New York alone rolled up a total of 93,297 cases of flu, 12,369 of pneumonia, and 12,356 deaths. The epidemic had reached our shores a month earlier when a crew of sailors landed at a southern port all suffering from the disease, and the Public Health Service in Washington later reported its rapid spread among the Army camps along the eastern seaboard. This world-wide epidemic—a pandemic—took the lives of nearly 25,000,000 people in 1918–1919.

As a student nurse at Presbyterian Hospital in New York, then at East 70th Street and Madison Avenue, I was assigned to 12-hour duty in a woman's "flu ward" and for six weeks I lived in the thick of the epidemic.

I wonder now how we stood it. We were always being urged to get outdoors during the day for fresh air and a change of scene but, for me, nothing compared to eight hours of solid sleep snatched from the sunshine, my eyes covered by a black silk stocking, my ears plugged with cotton. At the five o'clock alarm, I rose, showered, dressed, ate a large dinner and was back on the ward at seven. Those were dedicated weeks, as truly under fire as though we were with our brothers in the Argonne. Life was just one long emergency.

For me, nursing came alive during that test. In the preceding months at the school we had been steeped in theory, classes, and the meticulous practice of nursing techniques under close supervision. Technical proficiency had seemed all-important. Now, patients came first. Reassure them, ease them, help them, watch them, carry out every order, and comfort them. Their condition could change in split seconds. Our powers of observation sharpened. Our judgment dictated the call for a doctor. Theory and techniques must prove useful and helpful or we discarded them. This was nursing as I had dreamed of it; this was nursing at its most demanding. We grew to full professional stature in those dark nights.

DOROTHY DEMING, "RELIVING THE GREAT EPIDEMIC." OCTOBER 1957

"For backs that are taxing the nurse's ingenuity to keep from a bedsore I find nothing better than the unbeaten white of an egg patted over the area, and left untouched until it has dried. It forms almost a varnish, but a most comfortable and healing one. Stearate of zinc may be dusted on it before it dries to hasten the healing."

JANUARY 1923

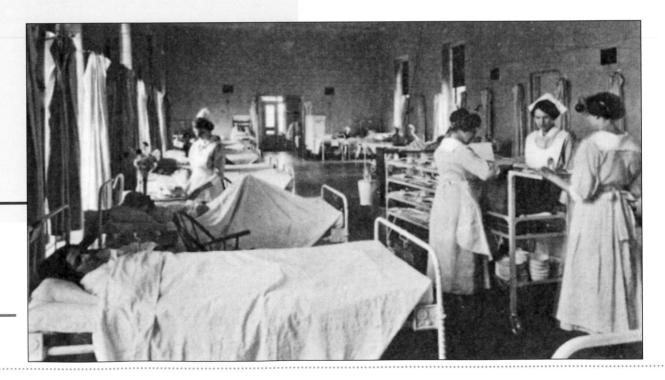

The wards of the Hartford Hospital.

But it was during the period of the epidemic last autumn that the schools met their greatest trials and sorrows. Wards were crowded with desperately ill patients, every department of the hospitals was handicapped because of the daily decrease of workers due to illness, and the nurses developed the disease every day. No hospital in the country could have met the difficulties without the assistance that came to them from every side. Nurses who had given up nursing work because of marriage or some other responsibility came back and took their places in the hospital wards. Women from every walk of life, nurses' aides, teachers, medical students, all came and offered their services and were given an opportunity to help. Women accustomed to hard work did whatever was necessary, assisted in the laundry, in the kitchen, washed dishes, swept, in short cared not what the task might be so long as they could help, so that the sick might be cared for.

In one hospital connected with a medical school, when the classes were of necessity discontinued, the students offered their services. The men went into the wards and served as orderlies and assistants to the nurses, carrying trays and helping in whatever way they could.

AUGUST 1919

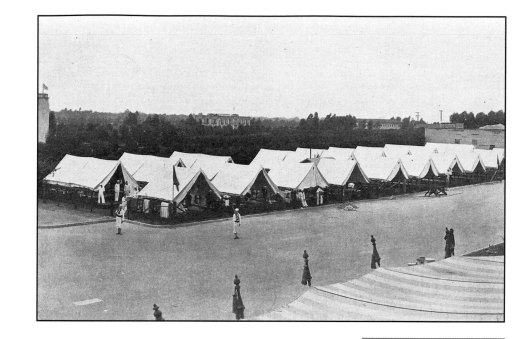

Isolation camp, San Diego, California.

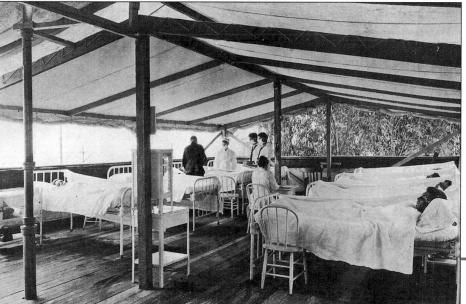

Pneumonia ward.

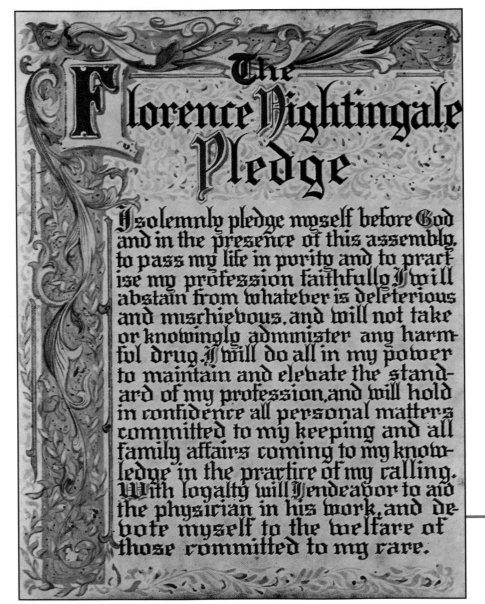

The Florence Nightingale Pledge

I solemnly pledge myself before God and in the presence of this assembly, to pass my life in purity and to practise my profession faithfully I will abstain from whatever is deleterious and mischievous, and will not take or knowingly administer any harmful drug. I will do all in my power to maintain and elevate the standard of my profession, and will hold in confidence all personal matters committed to my keeping and all family affairs coming to my knowledge in the practice of my calling. With loyalty will I endeavor to aid the physician in his work, and devote myself to the welfare of those committed to my care.

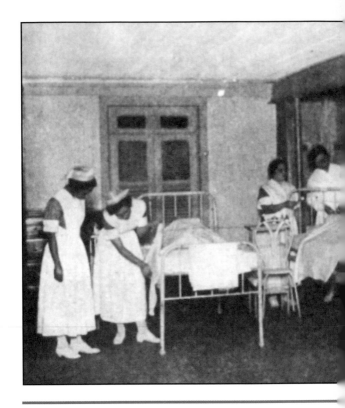

Teaching nurses in modern times.

The Nightingale Pledge was formulated by Lystra E. Gretter and a Committee for the Farrand Training School for Nurses, Detroit. It became a part of every nursing student's "capping."

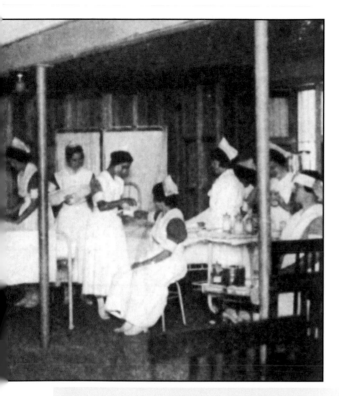

Professor of Nursing

*S*uch is the title recently bestowed on Effie J. Taylor by Yale University. The honor is unique, for Miss Taylor's subject is psychiatric nursing; indeed, we believe it is the first time that psychiatric nursing has been so dignified by any university . . .

An editorial writer of the New York Times, commenting on the appointment, wonders "what that excellent old nurse, Mrs. Sairey Gamp, would have said to a professorship of nursing."

JANUARY 1927

My Cap

*I*t lies here before me—a bit of white, crisp linen. There is nothing about it, visible to the eye, which makes it unique or at all prepossessing. An inanimate object, thirteen inches square, made from a large linen handkerchief—please use only the narrow-hemmed ones, says the prospectus—this, my cap.

It is something of a tyrant. It must always be laundered by my own hand because of its unhappy reaction to the ministrations of the laundry mangle. This is an exacting process, this laundering, and always demands doing on the nights I am weariest, and there could not possibly be a cap anywhere which shows so soon a bit of prolonged wear. It is full of temperament. It promptly proceeds to make its wearer look ridiculous if it gets pushed an infinitesimal part of an inch out of plumb. It becomes a sad and sorry affair, dejected and apologetic, if it ever meets a stray raindrop or a brisk breeze. Surely, 'tis not an easy cap to satisfy . . . Its shadow a slender spire beyond my head, preceding me down a dim hall in the hours of early morning or wavering a bit in a cold winter wind as I went home off duty in the evening, seemed alive with promises of the things I wanted to be.

It is the sign of my profession and tells of strong women and tender service. It tells of wise sympathy without sentimentality; broad understanding without cynicism; charity without weakness. By virtue of its own design it represents my training school . . .

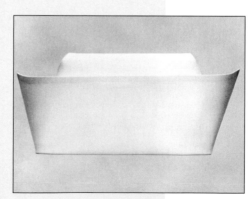

whose imprint will be a part of me for all the rest of my life. In strange places and under strange circumstances it is a tie with the dearly familiar.

FERN STUTZ, APRIL 1929

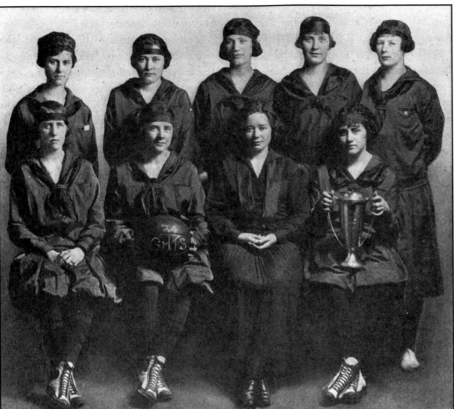

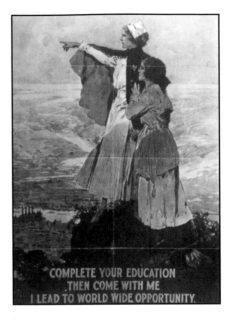

COMPLETE YOUR EDUCATION
THEN COME WITH ME
I LEAD TO WORLD WIDE OPPORTUNITY.

Grace Hospital basketball team,
Detroit, Michigan.

Metropolitan Hospital School of Nursing
Orchestra, Welfare Island, New York City.

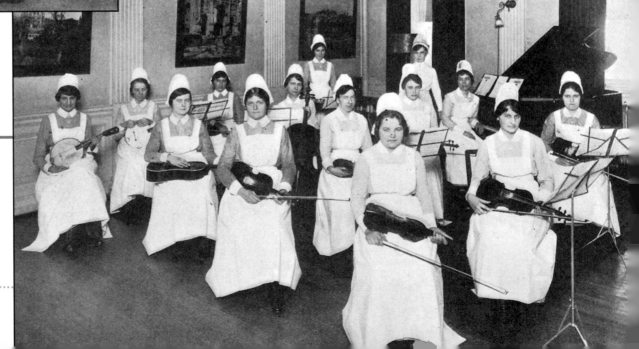

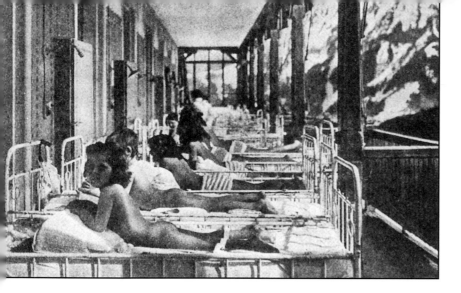

In Leysin, Switzerland, children with tuberculosis lie on a hospital porch, taking the sun cure (known as heliotherapy). American hospitals followed suit as tuberculosis sanitariums sprung up around the country.

It will be interesting to all our readers to know that the typhoid epidemic at the Sloane Maternity Hospital in New York which disabled so many doctors and nurses was finally traced to "Typhoid Mary," of world fame as a germ carrier, who had been employed as cook in the hospital, under an assumed name. This unfortunate woman is again segregated and is under treatment. A very disappointing feature of this epidemic was the apparent failure of anti-typhoid vaccine to protect all those who had been treated with it. The superintendent of the hospital writes that engaging a cook for an institution has become a hazardous undertaking.

MAY 1915

Dr.—, at the phone: "Please send the ethyl chloride to Ward II." Timid voice over the wire: "There is no one here by that name, doctor."

APRIL 1921

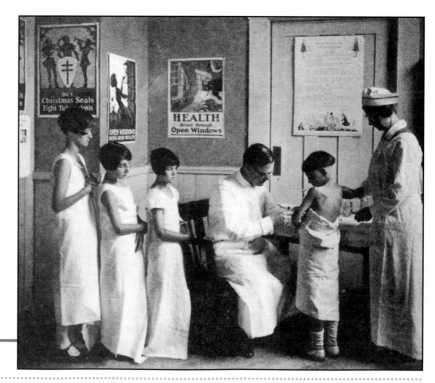

A tuberculin skin test clinic.

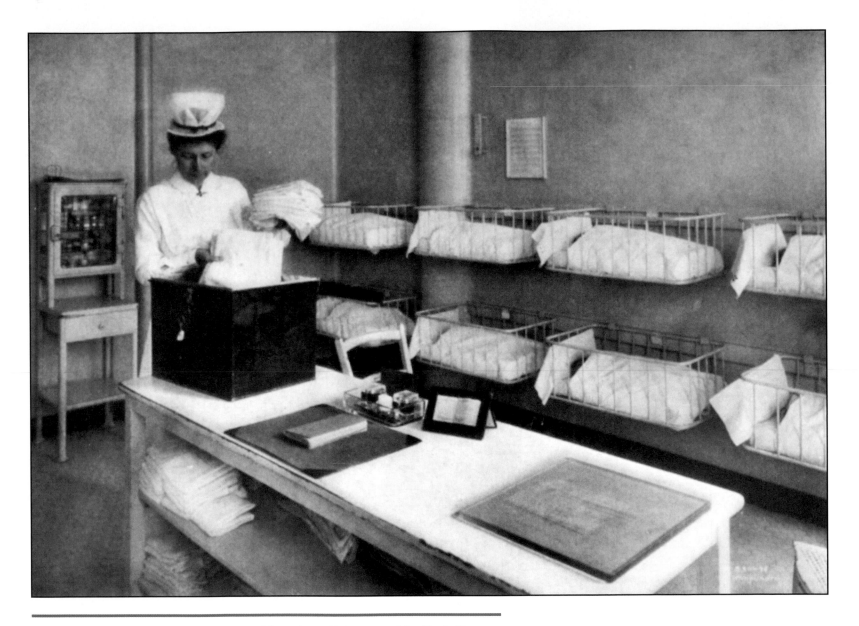

Folding diapers in the nursery at Manhattan Maternity and Dispensary, New York City.

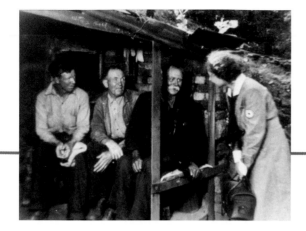

The Depression Years

1930–1939

The 1930s was a time of profound economic uncertainty. The decade brought sweeping changes in health care—changes that would dramatically alter the practice of nursing.

The stock market crash of 1929 resulted in the same serious unemployment for nurses as for the rest of the country, but for private duty nurses, it was devastating. There was a huge oversupply of nurses and few patients who could afford even the small fees they were charging. In 1932, the American Nurses Association launched a campaign to promote hospitals' hiring of graduate nurses for general duty work. The morale of these nurses was low, because they were seen as performing the tasks of students. In the depths of the depression, many nurses were willing to work in hospitals for room, board, and laundry.

The years of hardship made many nurses recognize the need for improvement in the education of nurses, the distribution of nursing services, and the welfare of those in the profession. In 1934, the final report of the Committee on the Grading of Nursing Schools gave impetus to these changes. In the decade of the thirties, 400 hospitals and 600 hospital nursing schools were closed.

The Social Security Act of 1935 proved to be extremely important legislation. It offered old-age benefits, unemployment assistance, maternal, child, and public health services, and training centers for "medical officers, graduate registered nurses, and public health sanitation personnel." It also authorized grants-in-aid to the states for the development and expansion of state and local health departments. By 1938, close to 25,000 public health nurses received stipends for postgraduate training. Unfortunately, however, the act excluded nonprofit hospital personnel from its compulsory old-age provisions and from unemployment compensation, the result of clever and successful lobbying by the hospital associations. This would not be remedied until the 1980s.

The decade is also remembered for milestones in health care and prevention. In the early 1930s, articles on the dangers of smoking were already appearing, which included the warning that smoking during pregnancy has a serious effect on the fetal heart rate. In addition, the discovery of sulfanilamide and its derivatives would change the practice of medicine.

Hospital insurance plans grew in tremendous popularity throughout the 1930s, which enabled people to pay their medical expenses and supplied a solution to the empty bed problem that could send hospitals into bankruptcy. As a result, new and more modern hospitals were being built. By the end of the decade, hospitals came to be seen as a necessary institution in every community, and nurses were a vital part of their operation.

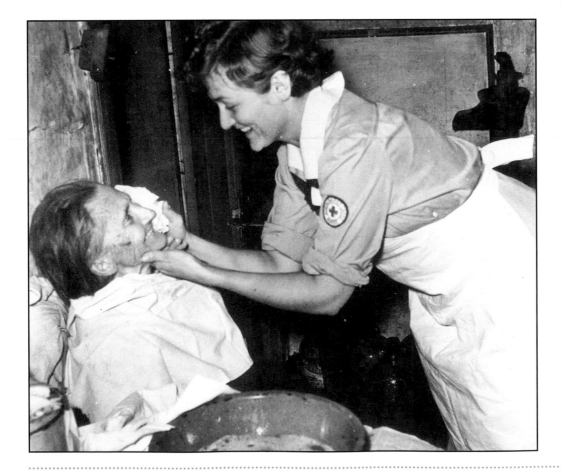

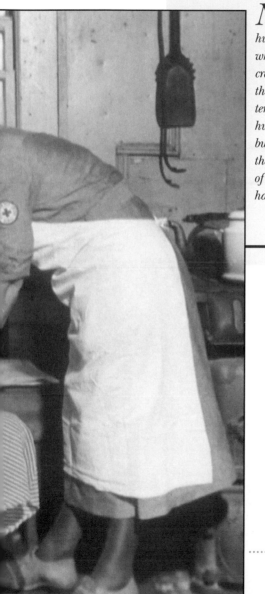

Effie J. Taylor on The Nature of Nursing

Nursing of all professions is a human profession and belongs to the whole world. It knows no color nor creed. It is for the poor as well as for the rich. Nursing is national and international in its relations, and every human being has a right to the contributions it can make. Its function is the conservation and the restoration of health for the perpetuation of a happy and a useful people.

MAY 1934

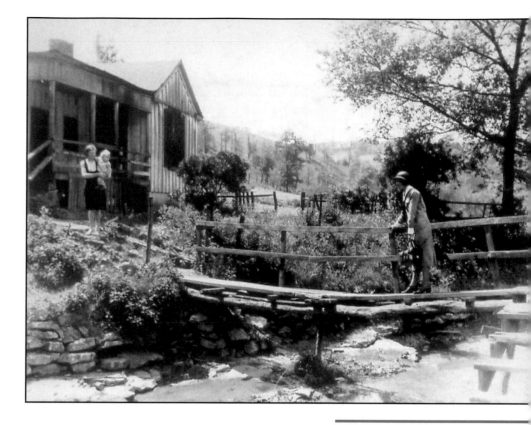

Daily trek across a West Virginia footbridge.

Letters

Dear Editor:

I am in the field of public health work and have found it very interesting and only wish I could do more, for the families are certainly most destitute out here. Food, such as milk, vegetables, and even fruit or potatoes would be a real treat for the children and parents who have had none for two years and more. I mean it, it is not a dream, believe me the fields and pastures are absolutely bare and Russian thistles have given feed for cattle and horses. We also are blessed with wind and dust.

May 1935

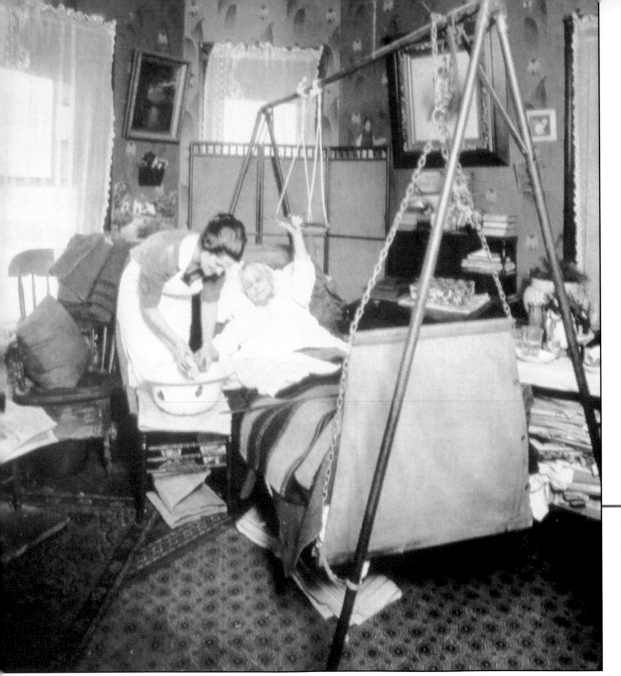

What Does the Public Expect From Nursing?

Nursing is changing its function; not its fundamental function of caring for those who need to be cared for, but perhaps we—the public—are expecting more than we used to expect from the nursing profession. I think today we expect two things. We expect not only the same skill and devotion which we have always counted on in this profession, but we also expect the nurse to act as teacher.

ELEANOR ROOSEVELT, JULY 1934

Boston visiting nurse bathing a patient in her home.

Baby care classes for boys.

Mealtime in pediatrics at Children's Memorial
Hospital, Chicago.

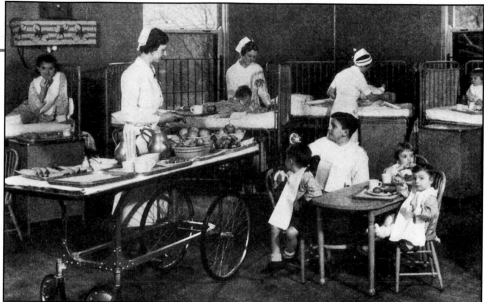

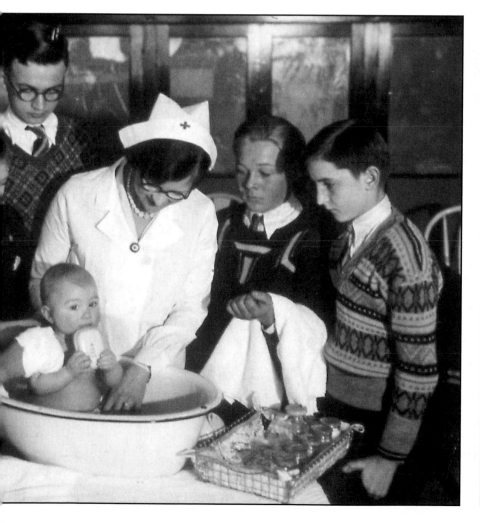

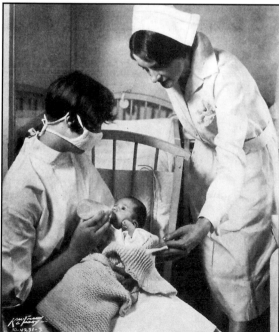

Teaching proper feeding
techniques to new mothers.

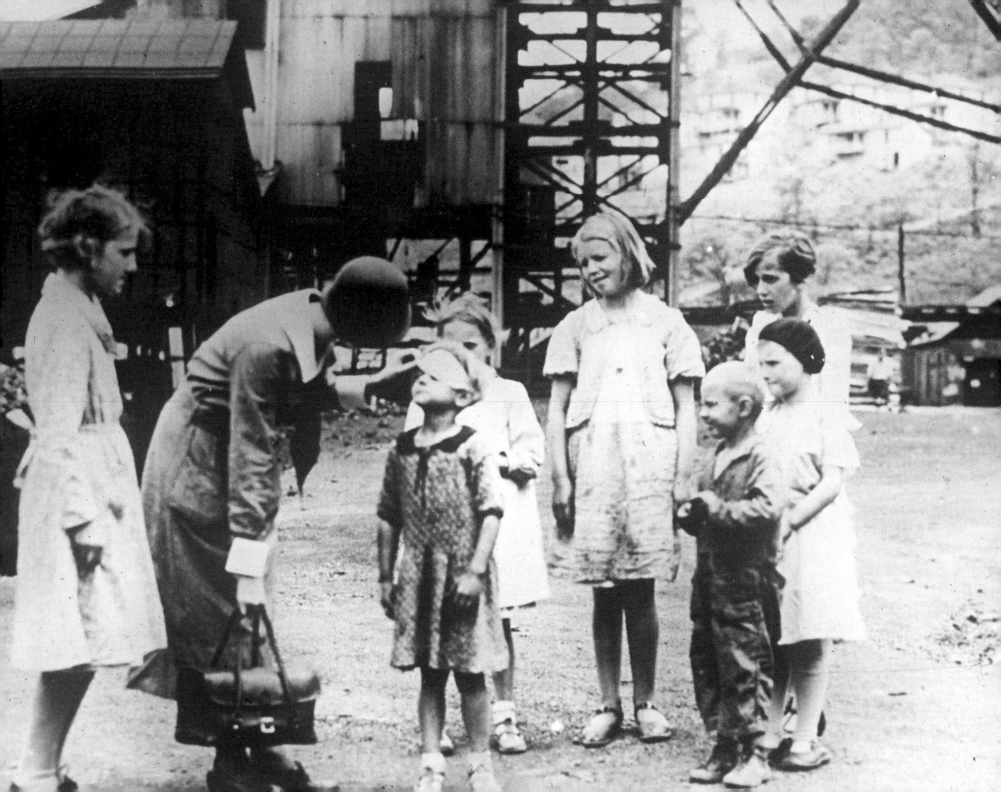

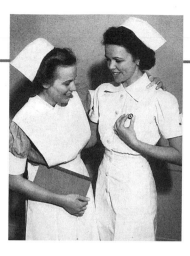

Commentary

Diane J. Mancino

The Journal's Student Pages

"Buried alive," "a prison sentence," and "the lost years," are some of the descriptions of nurses' training that appeared in the *American Journal of Nursing*'s Student Page. Becoming a permanent fixture in this publication in 1922 and continuing for fifty years, the monthly column, the Student Page, revealed what may seem today to be the extraordinary influence that nursing schools had over the lives of students. In the early days of nurses' training, students lived and worked at the hospital school for as long as three years. Isolated from their families as well as from non-nursing students, they depended on faculty and on each other for community life.

Early complaints led nursing superintendents to experiment with student government. Those in charge gradually gave students more responsibility over their schedules, first in planning social and recreational activities outside of school, such as basketball leagues, poetry readings, and drama clubs, and later as shared governance. One important way in which students found they could break through the insular walls of their training programs and develop a professional voice was in contributing to the Student Page.

Some of the most detailed accounts of nursing students' clinical experiences are recorded in the *Journal*'s Student Page. Student case studies examined prevalent communicable diseases such as tuberculosis, erysipelas, tetanus, measles, tularemia, yaws, poliomyelitis, anthrax, botulism, pemphigus neonatorum, rheumatic fever, and typhoid fever. In one example, Maysel Wagner, a student from Vanderbilt University School of Nursing in Nashville, Tennessee, authored "A Typhoid Case Summary" in the March 1927 issue of the *Journal*. In great detail, Wagner described the condition of five family members admitted to Vanderbilt Hospital, and how the lack of proper sanitation and personal hygiene in the home contributed to the disease:

"It was obvious that none of the family conformed to any rigid rules of sanitation. The patients' hands and nails were neglected, hair dirty, and their mouths were sore. This uncleanliness may be attributed to the poor means they had of washing. All the water had to be carried about sixty feet, from the spring, up an incline of 45 degrees. It had to be heated over a cooking stove. Baths were taken in a laundry tub and the face and hands cleansed in small tin basins. The family lived in a crude frame house with two rooms and a lean-to kitchen . . . A few feet below the house and about 50 feet above the spring was the open privy."

This student sample evidences thoughtful reflection on conditions in patients' lives that contribute to illness. Graduation speeches also occasionally appeared on the Student Page. A graduation address delivered during World War II by Pearl S. Buck to the Harlem School of Nursing class of 1943 strikes a special chord:

"I have never had the chance before, now that I think of it, to address a group of trained nurses as they are graduated from their school life and ready to begin their work with human beings . . . Whether you will be a good trained nurse or not, depends, for each of you, of course, upon the sort of person you are. All the training in the world will not make a good trained nurse of you if you are hard in your heart, selfish, and uncaring whether your patients live or die."

As early as 1910, the *Journal* carried articles about the development of student government in nursing schools. Beginning in 1922, the Student Page was also used to report on student experiences attending nurses' association meetings. In the 1940s, news about student organizations, along with lists of state student association presidents, began to appear. When the National Student Nurses Association (NSNA) was first organized in 1952, the *Journal* reported on annual student conventions in great detail, with photographs of board members and events.

As an example of an event sponsored by NSNA that was chronicled in the Student Page, in 1961, members embarked on a campaign to raise money

The amazing growth of schools of nursing, which have multiplied their number 143 times within the past fifty years, has come about not because the public wanted more nurses, but because the hospitals wanted more students. Hospitals run training schools for two reasons. The first reason is that it is cheaper to run a poor school than it is to employ graduate nurses. It is an extraordinary thing, but it seems to be a fact that hospitals regard the suggestion that they pay for their own nursing service as unreasonable. They have been receiving free service from students for so many years that they regard it as an inalienable right.

There is a real question whether the ordinary hospital can possibly afford to conduct a high grade nursing school.

It is still true that we are graduating each year 3,000 nurses so poorly educated that they would have difficulty in getting positions in a good department store. These are not the type of young women whom we really want to have taking full responsibility for life or death in the sick room.

(From Nursing Schools Today and Tomorrow, *the final report of the Committee on Grading Nursing Schools.)*

MAY 1930

By the 1930s, collegiate education was getting serious attention. Beginning in 1909, when the school of nursing at the University of Minnesota was organized under the university rather than under a hospital, a number of institutions offered a four- or five-year combined diploma and baccalaureate program.

The Yale School of Nursing, which opened in 1924, was the first to be established as a separate university department with its own budget and its own dean, Annie W. Goodrich. It accepted only students who had completed two years of college, and then provided them with a 28-month course leading to a Bachelor of Nursing degree. The program was funded by a five-year grant from the Rockefeller Foundation, which also helped to fund a similar program at Vanderbilt University, under the direction of Shirley Titus.

to build a new nursing student dormitory in Taipei, after learning that existing conditions were deplorable. Within three years, $34,000 U.S. dollars were collected through the efforts of 50 state student associations selling shares in the Student Nurses' Dormitory for twenty-five cents apiece. By March 1966, the dormitory, fully furnished and equipped with visual aids, books, and educational materials, was dedicated. Other issues taken up in the Student Page in the 1960s and 1970s included racism, minority recruitment, and civil rights. Through the years, the *Journal*'s Student Page gave students an opportunity to grow as professionals and to organize in strength.

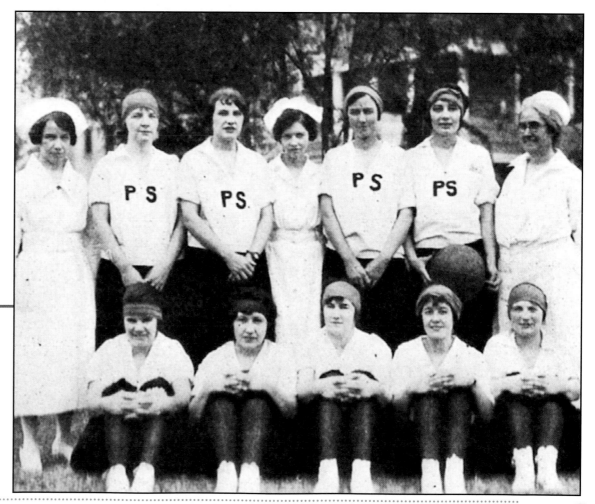

Extracurricular activity. The basketball team at Physicians and Surgeons Hospital School of Nursing, San Antonio, with their coaches.

A Delano nurse making her rounds on a Maine coastal island. The Delano Red Cross Nursing Service was established from funds set aside by Jane A. Delano, Director of Red Cross Nursing during World War I, in her will as a memorial to her parents. It provided funding to pay for public health nurses in remote areas where public health nursing services were not readily available.

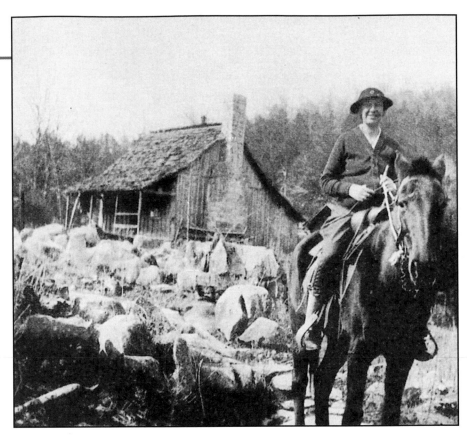

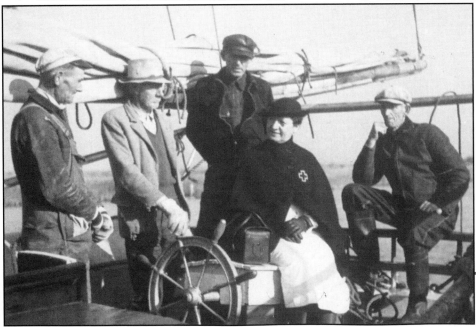

A Delano nurse travelling by schooner to Smith Island, Maryland.

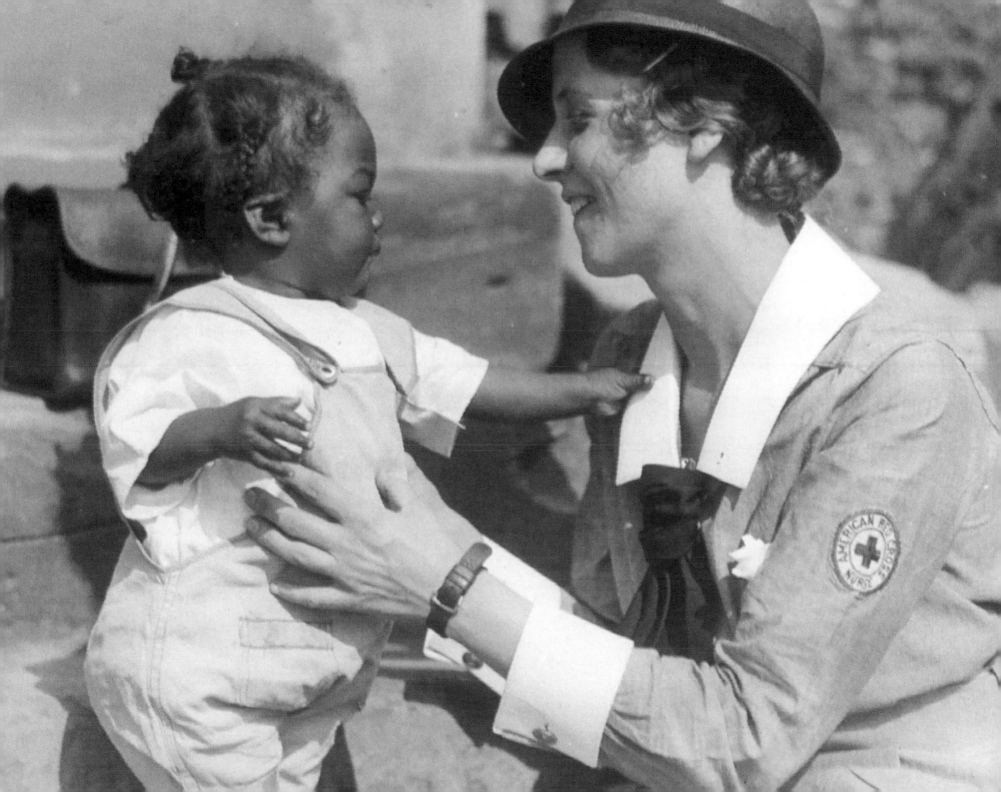

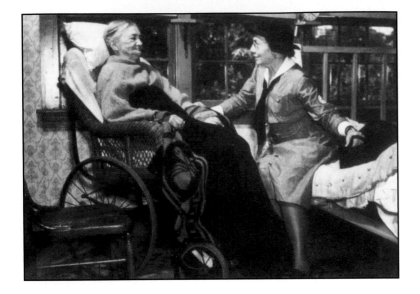

During fiscal year 1937–1938, public health nurses made more than one million visits to the sick.

Principal Causes of Death in 1939

*N*ever before has there been even a close approach to the figures of 1939 for these four diseases: measles, scarlet fever, whooping cough, and diphtheria. The death rate for the group was 4.2 per 100,000, marking a drop of 34 per cent in a single year and of 79 per cent in ten years; and each individual disease fell to a new minimum.

Tuberculosis recorded fewer than 45 deaths per 100,000 insured lives in 1939. This is a decline in rate of 4.9 per cent in a year. . . .

The decline in the pneumonia death rate of 15.2 per cent in a single year is probably the most striking development of 1939 in the entire field of public health. The death rate has dropped 52 per cent in ten years.

The cancer death rate rose for the third successive year and reached a new high of 101 per 100,000. Nineteen thirty-nine was the first year in which the rate exceeded 100. The crude death rate from cancer has increased 30 per cent in ten years.

There was another sharp rise in 1939 in the mortality rate for coronary artery diseases. These conditions now rank high in the list of causes of death, and the death rate in 1939 (40.2 per 100,000) was almost nine times that recorded at the beginning of the decade just closed.

The death rate from diabetes in 1939 was 27.5 per 100,000, as compared with 24.8 in 1938.

MARCH 1940

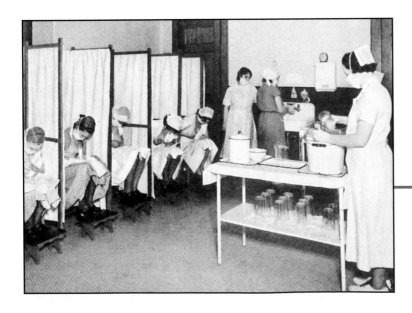

The milk room, Mothers' Milk Bureau, Children's Welfare Association, New York City, where breast milk donations were collected under careful supervision.

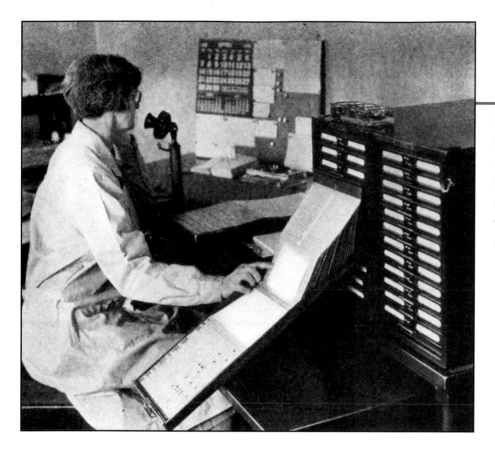

Registrar in the Nurses' Official Registry of Minneapolis. District nurses' associations took over the work of hospital and alumnae registries and used the title "official" to identify and differentiate themselves from the proliferation of commercial registries. In 1930, the American Nurses Association was doing a comprehensive study of registries that would culminate in a set of minimum standards.

Nurses' House in Babylon, New York was a place nurses could go for rest and convalescence. It was donated in 1924 by Emily Bourne as a way of expressing her thanks for the excellent nursing care given to members of her family. In 1960, it was sold to the Roman Catholic Diocese of Rockville Center and the proceeds put into an investment portfolio that continues to provide assistance to nurses in need.

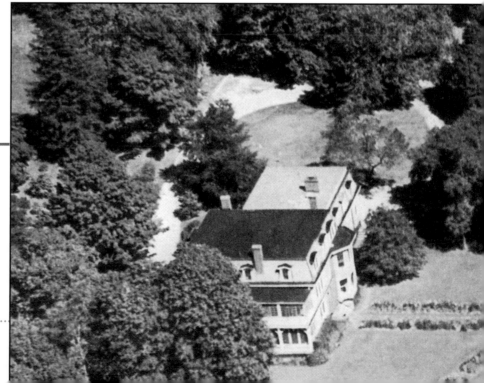

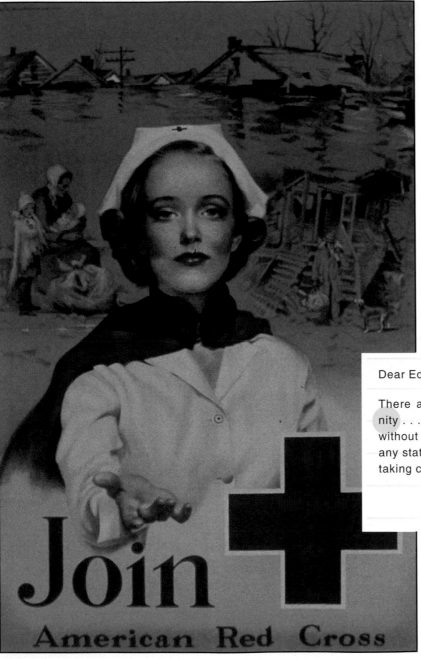

Join
American Red Cross

Women's Earnings

A study conducted by the Women's Bureau during 1931 showed that "trained nurses with less than five years experience had median earnings of $1,650. Teachers and secretaries did not average this until after ten years experience, and the bookkeeper and stenographer groups did not approximate this median until after fifteen years experience."

DECEMBER 1934

Letters

Dear Editor:

There are many nurses who still think California the land of opportunity . . . Wandering nurses who come to the state without an RN, and without evidence of membership in the American Nurses Association in any state, but add to the burden of the nurses of the state association in taking care of the surplus nurses who are now there.

November 1931

Letters

Dear Editor:

While we are anxious to be of assistance to our own unemployed, we do not wish to have any more out of state nurses coming here and would like to have you publish a statement to that effect. There is not sufficient work for nurses who have always lived here [in Alabama] and while we do not wish to appear inhospitable, frankly speaking for the good of the profession, we would like to have them remain away.

March 1934

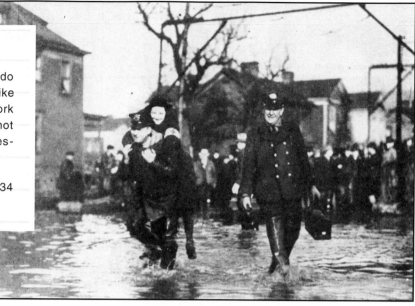

Police officers carried the nurse and her supply bag across a flooded street during the Ohio-Mississippi flood of 1937.

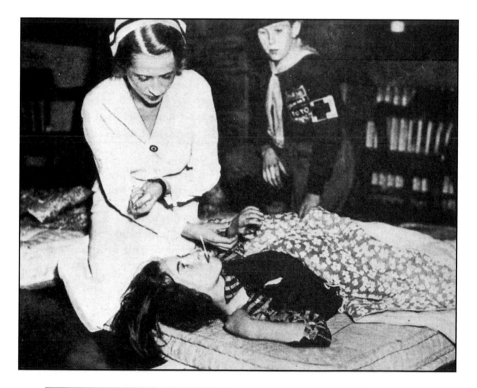

Wheeling, West Virginia flood sufferer.

"Eight-hour duty, the dream of all private duty nurses, has at last come true for us in St. Louis. There does not seem to have ever been a time when shortening the hours of the private duty nurse has not been a subject near the hearts of all of us, but eight hours seemed the all but impossible Mecca. Now we are actually experiencing it and finding the results as splendid as any of us ever hoped for."

MAY 1934

Letters

Christmas 1939

The scent of balsam—crimson holly berries—shining Christmas trees—candles giving themselves in light—carol singing—happy children—the gaiety of crowds in the streets.

And the shadow of a world at war.

But Christmas is too old a festival, too bound up with our lives and traditions to be lightly set aside because of war. Christmas is the feast of Peace.

We, who have chosen nursing, have thereby allied ourselves with those other groups of professional people who, with us, have the very seeds of peace in their keeping. For the healing of mankind—its physical, mental, emotional, spiritual wounds—must surely lead to the healing of the nations.

Nurses, moreover, the world around, are bound together by friendships, hopes, aspirations, and purposes.

Our wish for us all this Christmas is that the priceless bonds between us may be strengthened so that an indestructible and creative force—Nursing—may be used to help restore this world to Peace.

—The Editors
December 1939

Dear Editor:

Miss Nutting certainly started something when she began collecting and compiling nursing history.

I submit that history should not be studied; it should only be read. There might be a few hours of required reading, with general discussion afterwards. The good of history is in its lessons for life. It is useless to memorize a lot of names, dates, and places.

L. L. Dock
June 1931

Three Red Cross public health nurses head out on another day visiting patients during a typhoid epidemic in Kentucky in 1935.

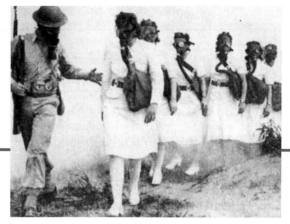

Days of Infamy
and a New Era

1940–1949

On December 7, 1941, which President Franklin D. Roosevelt called "a day that will live in infamy," the Japanese bombed the U.S. Navy base at Pearl Harbor. On December 8, the United States and Great Britain declared war on Japan, and on December 11, Germany and Italy declared war on the United States. During World War II, 292,131 Americans were killed and almost 670,000 were injured. Throughout this time, nurses were called upon in mass numbers to serve their country.

With the rise of Hitler and the German conquest of country after country in Europe, most Americans had known war was inevitable. In July 1940, the Nursing Council for National Defense was formed. Its mission was to make the best use of existing nursing resources to meet military and civilian needs. A tall order, this involved assisting the Red Cross with its enrollment of nurses into the Army and Navy Nurse Corps; updating training for inactive nurses so they could go back to work; increasing enrollment in nursing schools; and enlisting the help of volunteers and auxiliary workers.

The demand for nurses was acutely felt on the battlefields and at home. Although military service seemed more dramatic, the needs on the home front intensified as civilian hospitals lost personnel, as defense plants required a nurse presence, and as public health nurses were recruited from their normal posts. To no surprise, there was a dire need for an increase in student enrollment. In order to deal with the crisis, in 1943, the U.S. Cadet Nurse Corps was formed. A government-subsidized nursing training program, the corps provided 123,000 nurses for the cause.

Despite these efforts, there was still a nursing shortage. American troops in war zones were suffering heavy casualties. On January 6, 1945, in his State of the Union message, President Roosevelt called for a draft of nurses. Soon after, the Nurses Selective Service Act of 1945 began moving through Congress. The American Nurses Association, the National League for Nursing Education, and the National Organization for Public Health Nursing endorsed the principle of a draft of nurses as a first step to a draft of all women. It proved, however, to be unnecessary; nurses responded overwhelmingly to this call and the end of the war now seemed imminent. By September 2, 1945, the formal end of the war, 31.1 percent of all active professional nurses had served with the Armed Forces.

Even when the war was over, the nursing scarcity was still a problem. While in the military, nurses experienced a level of autonomy and respect that they did not feel back home. Many nurses returning from military service no longer wanted to work in traditional hospital settings, where professional esteem and salaries were low.

Delegates to the ANA's 1946 convention knew these problems had to be immediately addressed. As a first step, they voted to adopt an economic security program with the state nurses associations acting as the nurses' representatives in collective bargaining with employers. Despite these and other measures, at the close of the decade, few women were choosing to enter the nursing field.

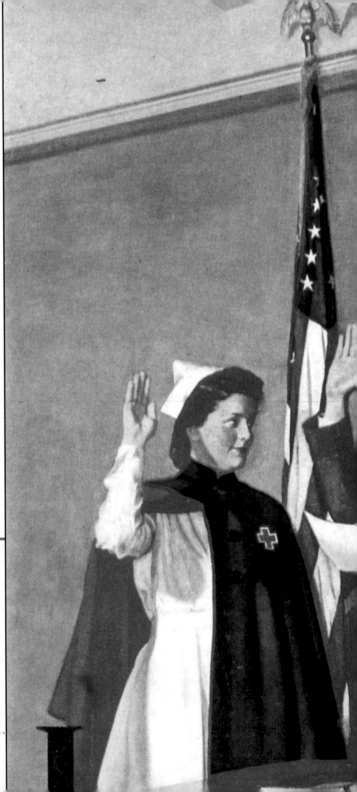

I do solemnly swear that I will support and defend the Constitution of the United States against all enemies, foreign and domestic; that I will bear true faith and allegiance to the same; that I take this obligation freely, without any mental reservation or purpose of evasion; and that I will well and faithfully discharge the duties of the office on which I am about to enter. So help me, God.

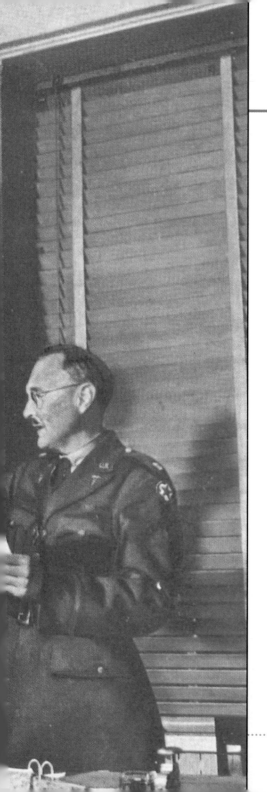

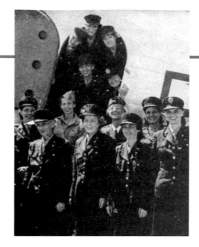

Commentary

Julia Plotnick

Nursing and the Military

The military has always had a large impact on society—shaping economics, politics, and the health care system. Nursing is just one profession that has evolved, in part, through interaction with the military over the course of the twentieth century. A number of key developments took place during the First and Second World Wars that have had a lasting impact on the field.

When the United States entered the First World War, military and civilian authorities realized there was an acute shortage of trained nurses. In response to this situation, the Vassar Training Camp and the Army School of Nursing were launched in 1918. The camp was designed to raise the number of nurses in general, whereas the school was specifically geared toward increasing the number of nurses in military service. In the final analysis, both programs served to increase the level of professionalism and expertise of new nurses.

At the onset of U.S. involvement in the Second World War, there was once again the realization on the part of military and civilian leadership that nursing education and training programs would have to be expanded. In 1940, the Nursing Council for National Defense was established in order to conduct a national inventory of registered nurses and determine the role of nursing in the national defense system. After war was declared, this organization was renamed the National Nursing Council for War Services, and worked toward increasing enrollments in nursing schools.

As the war progressed, it became apparent that increased funding would be required if the military's need for expanded and improved nursing education would be met. Thus, the Appropriations Act of 1942 set a new precedent by including funds for nursing education. In 1943, the Nurse Training Act was passed. This included a $60-million appropriation for nursing education and resulted in the formation of the U.S. Cadet Nurse Corps. Ultimately, the combination of federal appropriations and the Cadet Nurse Corps would lead to significant improvements in the standards of nursing education, for in order to receive federal funding, a nursing program had to demonstrate that it met NLNE requirements.

The ability of the military and the nursing fields to benefit mutually from their interrelationship stems from a variety of sources, including the civilian-controlled democratic system of government in the United States, and the trend (since the war of 1812) toward increased military professionalism. Traditionally, the government has been wary of stretching the military's mandate beyond that of territorial national defense. When a demand for nursing expertise arose, the response was not to expand military nursing, but, rather, to look toward more efficient civilian nursing programs to fill the need.

The interaction between nursing and the military in the United States has, to a large degree, proven beneficial to both parties. In times of conflict, the military has created a demand for nursing expertise and provided the means to pay for it. Nursing leaders, on their part, have seized the opportunities offered by increased military demand, and used them to widen and professionalize nursing education and to enhance the prestige of the field. This has led to the enhancement not only of American military nursing, but also of the nursing profession in general.

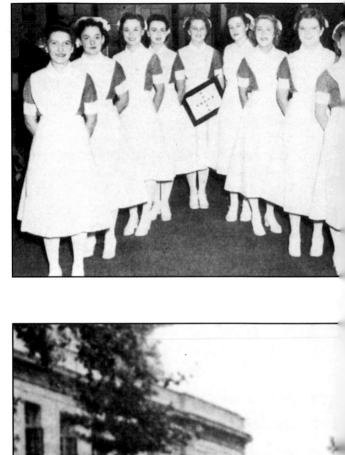

Senior student nurses leaving the Pan American building, Washington, DC, in 1942, after having been enrolled in the first Red Cross student nurse reserve group formed in the United States. These young women who are about to become graduate nurses pledged their future to Uncle Sam and will become available for active duty in the Army and Navy.

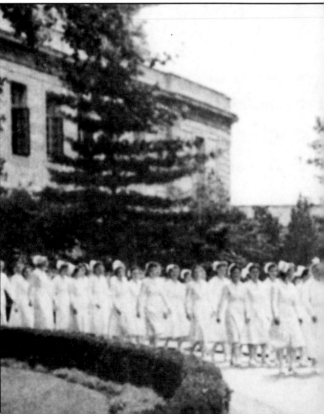

The June 1943 class of the M. B. Johnson School of Nursing, Elyria, Ohio, exhibiting the service flag for 100 percent senior class enrollment in the Red Cross Student Reserve.

Letters

Dear Editor:

Don't look back from a dull middle age and think "And I had a chance to experience the unusual and didn't take it!" Young nurses have grand opportunities right now, through enlistment in the Army or the Navy Nurse Corps, for unusual experiences which seldom come when conditions are normal. Live venturously *now*. We who served in the Army and Navy during the World War are *so* thankful that *we got up and went.*

Two Old Nurses, New York.
March 1941

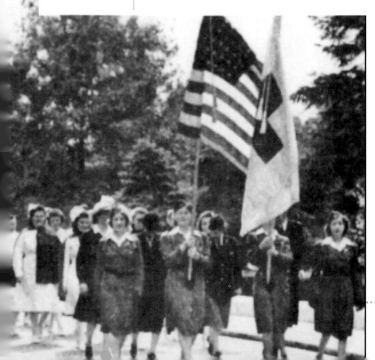

This appealing poster, in the national colors, was widely used in connection with the recruitment of student nurses and was sent with a covering letter to all colleges admitting women.

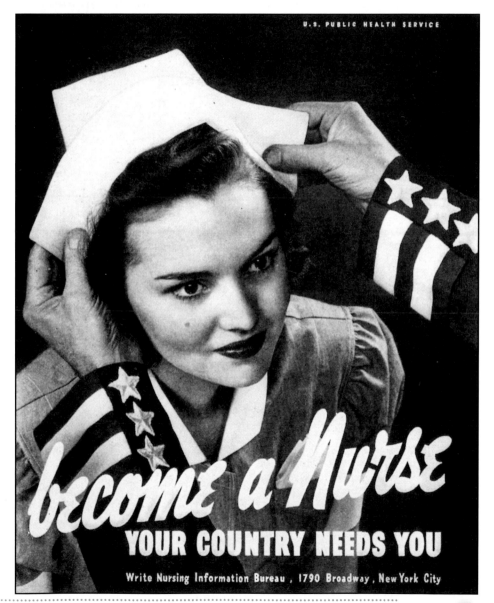

U.S. PUBLIC HEALTH SERVICE

become a Nurse
YOUR COUNTRY NEEDS YOU
Write Nursing Information Bureau, 1790 Broadway, New York City

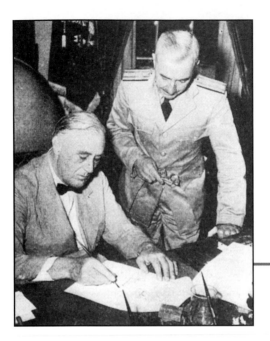

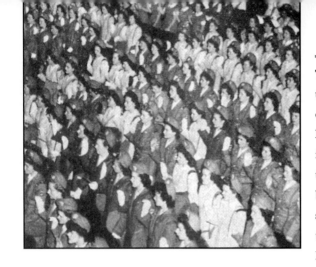

National induction of cadet nurses in San Francisco.

President Roosevelt affixes his signature to the Bolton Bill, while Dr. Thomas Parran, Surgeon General, USPHS, witnesses the signing.

The U.S. Cadet Nurse Corps was created by federal law in 1943 to fill the country's enormous need for nurses, both civilian and military, during World War II. That law was the Bolton Act (introduced by Rep. Frances Payne Bolton of Ohio). The Bolton Act provided funds for a massive public relations campaign to recruit nursing students; to cover the cost of all educational expenses, including tuition, books, a uniform designed by couturier Molly Parnis, and a monthly stipend for students admitted to the 1,125 participating schools; and to support educational activities that strengthened the schools. A new Division of Nurse Education was established within the U.S. Public Health Service (USPHS) to administer the program under the direction of the dynamic Lucile Petry. By 1948, when the last Cadet Corps students were graduated, $161 million dollars had been spent, but the effect of the Corps on nursing standards was far reaching, making education out of what had been training.

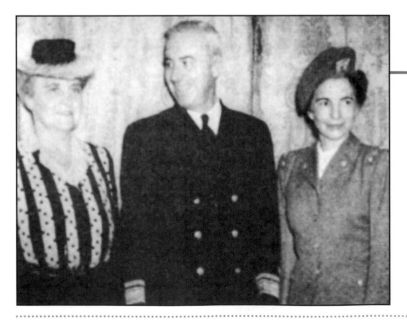

In Washington: Representative Frances P. Bolton; Dr. Thomas Parran, Surgeon General, USPHS; and Lucile Petry, Director, U. S. Cadet Nurse Corps.

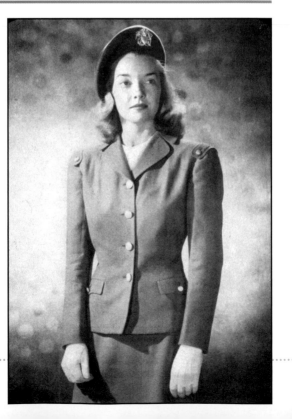

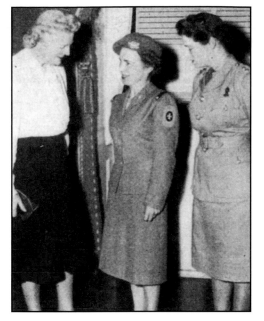

Lucile Petry, Director, U.S. Cadet Nurse Corps, wearing the official new Cadet Nurse Corps uniform, called on Mrs. Winston Churchill and Subaltern Mary Churchill at the White House. Both Mrs. Churchill and Miss Churchill exclaimed over the new uniform.

Japanese evacuee nurse assists new evacuee family in the internment camp.

NURSE STEWARDESSES

In the 1930s, major airlines, including American and United Airlines, began using registered nurses as in-flight personnel to assist passengers and to be available to handle in-flight emergencies. A nursing background became a prerequisite for employment. With the nursing shortage during World War II, these requirements were relaxed, although American Airlines instead required stewardess candidates to possess a college education.

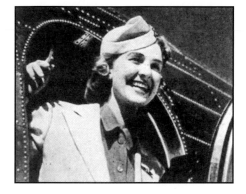

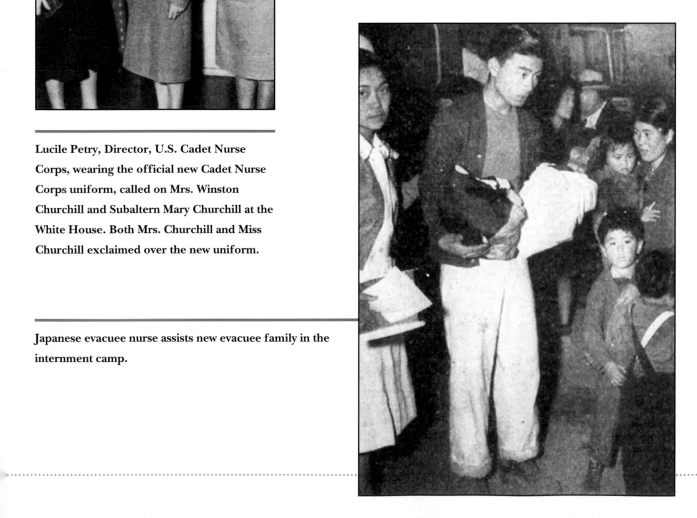

The shameful internment of more than 100,000 Americans of Japanese ancestry found *AJN* succumbing to the propaganda of the War Relocation Authority. Calling the victims "evacuees" and the internment camps "pioneer communities," *AJN* in 1943 reported that the evacuee nurses worked tirelessly in the project hospitals for $19 a month, the salary established for professionals by the War Relocation Authority. Student nurses taken by the evacuation order from their schools of nursing also worked in the project hospitals, although many were able to finish in schools that were willing to accept students of Japanese ancestry because of the efforts of the National Nursing Council for War Service and the National Student Relocation Council.

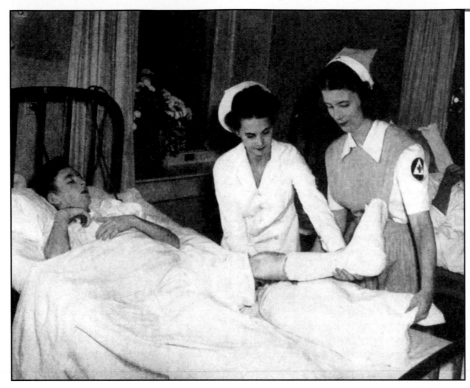

With nurses in short supply, the Red Cross initiated a Volunteer Nurse's Aide Corps to fill in where nursing services were needed.

Mayor Fiorello LaGuardia, New York City, signing a proclamation urging registered nurses to enroll in the first reserve of the Red Cross for service with the Army and Navy.

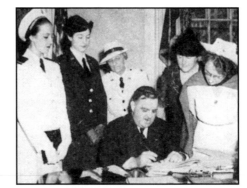

On November 28, 1942, the readiness of the home front for disaster was tested when Boston's Cocoanut Grove nightclub became a fiery holocaust, killing half of the 800 people packed inside. Hospitals went into disaster mode; doctors and nurses reported immediately and patients flooded in needing treatment for shock and for flash burns, anoxemia, and inhaled smoke and flames.

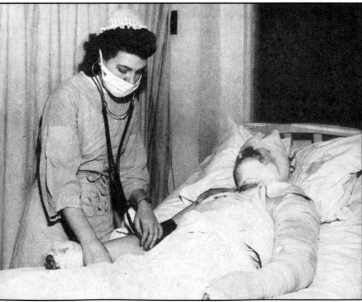

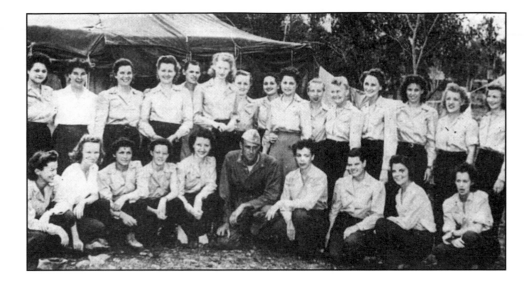

The first contingent of Army nurses in an aerial evacuation unit operating on Guadalcanal. They cared for wounded soldiers being flown from combat zones to station hospitals.

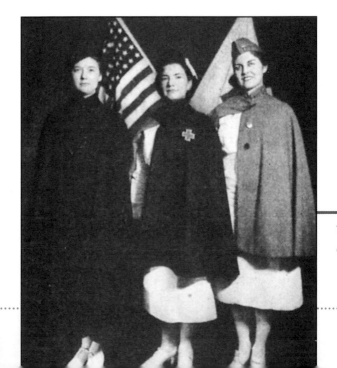

Uniforms of the Navy, Red Cross, and Army nurses.

A State of War Exists

*A*merican men, women, and children have been killed by enemy action.

American nurses are needed now in great numbers to care for the armed forces and to relieve the suffering of helpless people in hospitals, in air raid shelters, and in the evacuation line of "target" cities. All American men and women will be listed for service to our country. Many thousand more nurses are needed to perform services which only the professional nurse can give.

American nurses have never failed to respond to our country's call for help. We shall not fail now.

If you are a graduate of a school meeting Red Cross requirements, if your health is good, if you are not over fifty years of age, apply today for enrollment in the national nursing reserve of the Red Cross.

MARY BEARD, DIRECTOR,
AMERICAN RED CROSS NURSING SERVICE
JANUARY 1942

*"P*assage of the bill for commissioned rank for Army nurses, signed by the President and so made law on June 22, 1944, was preceded by the bill granting commissioned rank to Navy nurses, which was signed on February 26."

North Africa, 1942.

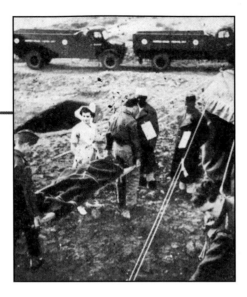

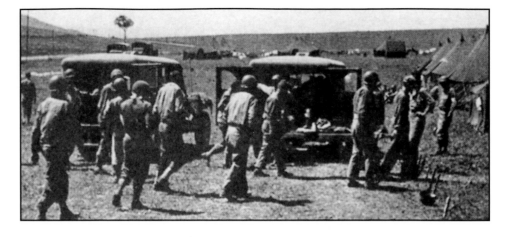

The first ambulances to arrive at this evacuation hospital in North Africa shortly after a battle.

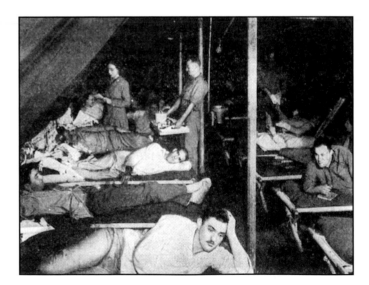

Army nurses and corpsmen care for wounded soldiers in a ward tent in North Africa.

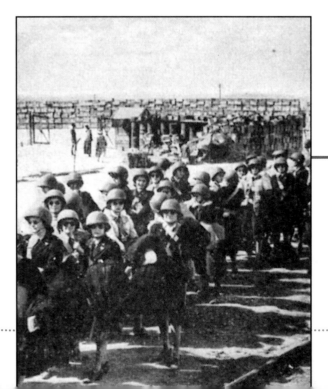

U. S. Army nurses arrive on the East African Front.

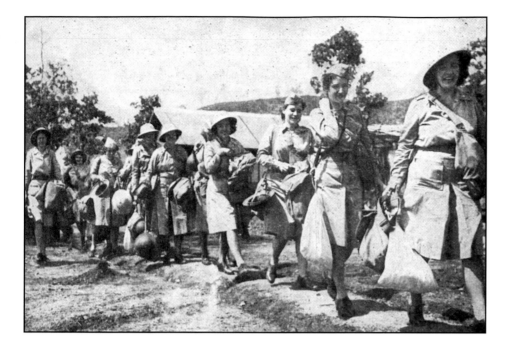

The first contingent of U.S. Army nurses to be sent to an Allied advanced base in New Guinea.

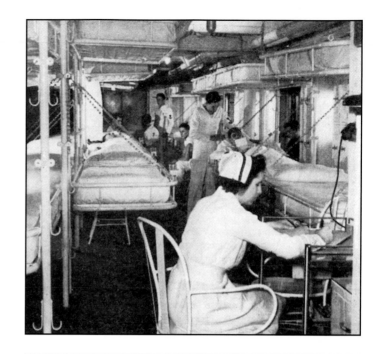

Patients, corpsmen, and Navy nurse in a medical ward on the USS *Solace*. Empty beds are raised up and secured.

"The nurses lived like the soldiers. There was no heat nor hot water for bathing. There was no light, but that from a candle, a flashlight, or a lantern in the pyramidal tents where they lived, four and six in a group. They had cots on which to place their bed rolls. They could never expect to unpack completely. In their off-duty time they washed their heavy herringbone twill slack suits, and it was a constant problem to dry them in the cold and rainy weather. They stood in line for their food, to wash their mess kits, and often when they ate.

The work was exhausting. The period of duty was often longer than twelve hours, and fatigue was increased from bending constantly over the low Army cots that stood scarcely eighteen inches from the ground. It took a great deal of energy to pull four-buckle overshoes out of the mud at every step all day long. The patients were very ill, and each nurse had a great number to care for."

VINCOE PAXTON, ANC
FEBRUARY 1945

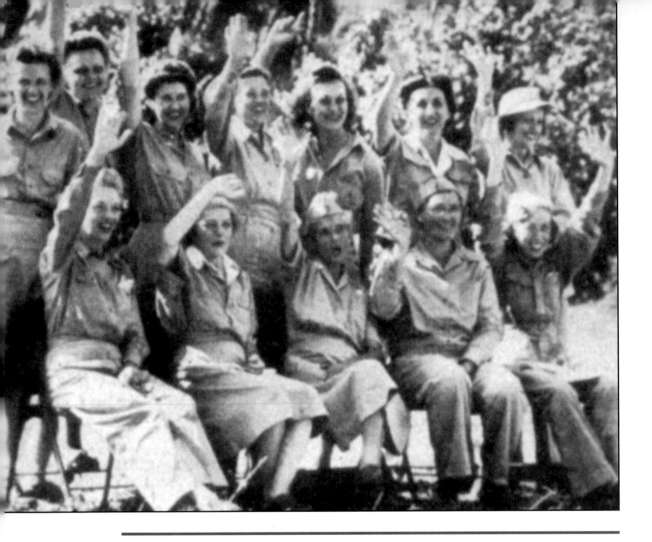

Army nurses just liberated from Santo Tomás internment camp in the Philippines.

Sixty-six Army nurses serving in the Philippines were held as POWs for 37 months in Japanese camps. This internment followed months of courageous duty under fire from advancing Japanese troops after the fall of Manila, Bataan, and Corregidor. The wartime movie *So Proudly We Hail* starring Claudette Colbert was based on their experiences.

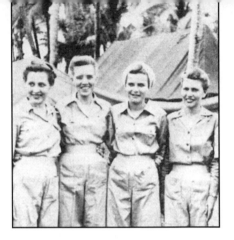

Four of the liberated nurses after they arrived on Leyte.

"*E*tched in my mind forever are the scenes that I saw in the field hospitals in Bataan and in the tunnel hospital in Corregidor. Working day in and day out, the doctors and nurses in Bataan and Corregidor did not know what rest meant, and they suffered along with the soldiers on the front all the privations and the hardships that made the resistance offered by the Filipinos and Americans in the Philippines an epic that has passed into immortality . . . They had gone without food, they had suffered the agony and the torture of homesickness, loneliness, and despair in the jungles of Bataan, they had been under continuous shell and fire for days on end, but they did not falter and they gave of themselves without stint."

LT. COL. CARLOS ROMULO,
a member of Douglas MacArthur's staff
AUGUST 1942

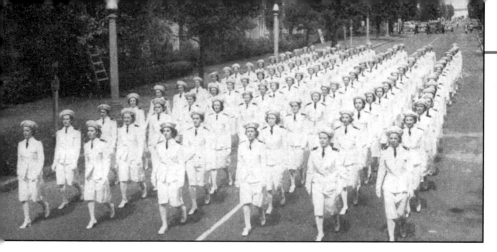

Navy nurses, San Diego.

The most enthusiastic letters the editors receive are from nurses in service who have triumphantly adjusted to the amazing gamut of military nursing experiences. And why wouldn't they? Nursing takes on a new importance when they realize that the injured "are so perfectly sure they will recover as soon as they hear that nurses are in the vicinity."

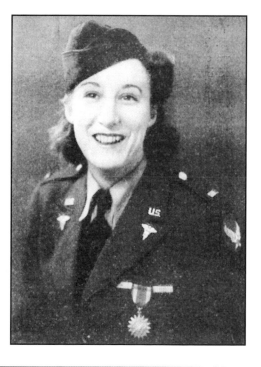

Lt. Elsie S. Ott, RN, wearing the first Air Medal ever awarded a woman.

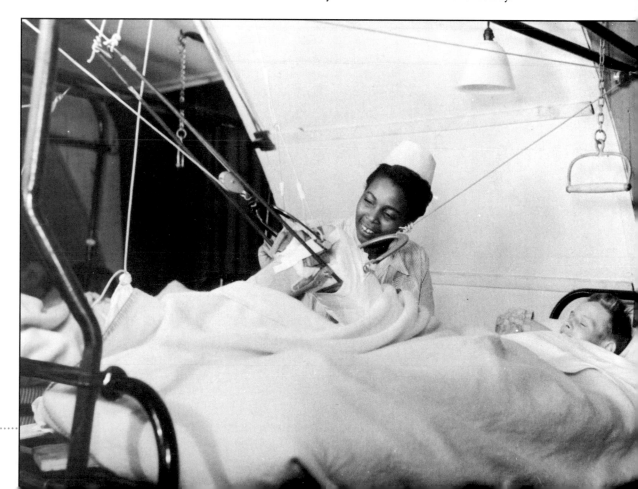

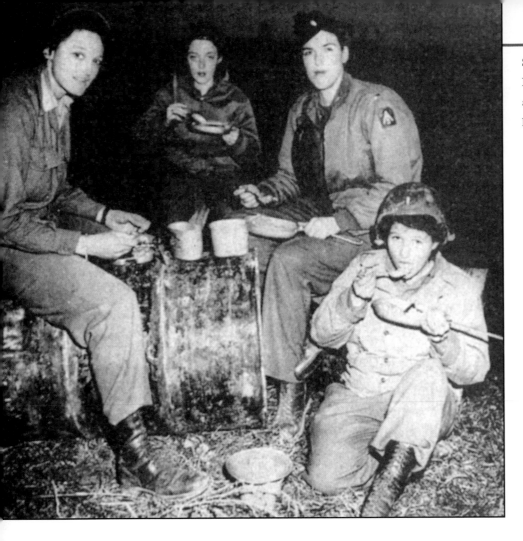

Some of the first Army nurses to land on the Anzio-Nettuno beachhead. Recovered from their seasickness, after a trip in a tossing LCI, they are eating their first hot meal.

"The unit arrived in the harbor on D-day-plus-three. They ran into trouble right off—bad weather, a breakdown on one of the ships, and enemy raids on harbor and beach. The trip had been a rough one, during which the convoy was attacked by German dive bombers fourteen times in thirty-six hours. As the small LCI on which the nurses traveled was badly tossed about, twenty-two of them were hauled by ropes onto a larger LST from which they made the landing on the fifth day after the invasion. The other thirty nurses were so seasick that their landing was deferred until D-day-plus-six."

FREDERICK CLAYTON
MAY 1944

Army nurses disembarking from a landing craft in Naples harbor.

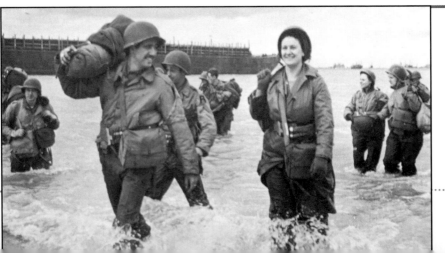

U.S. Army nurses and members of the Army Medical Corps arriving at the Normandy beachhead wade ashore from their landing craft. They are on their way to field hospitals to care for wounded Allied soldiers.

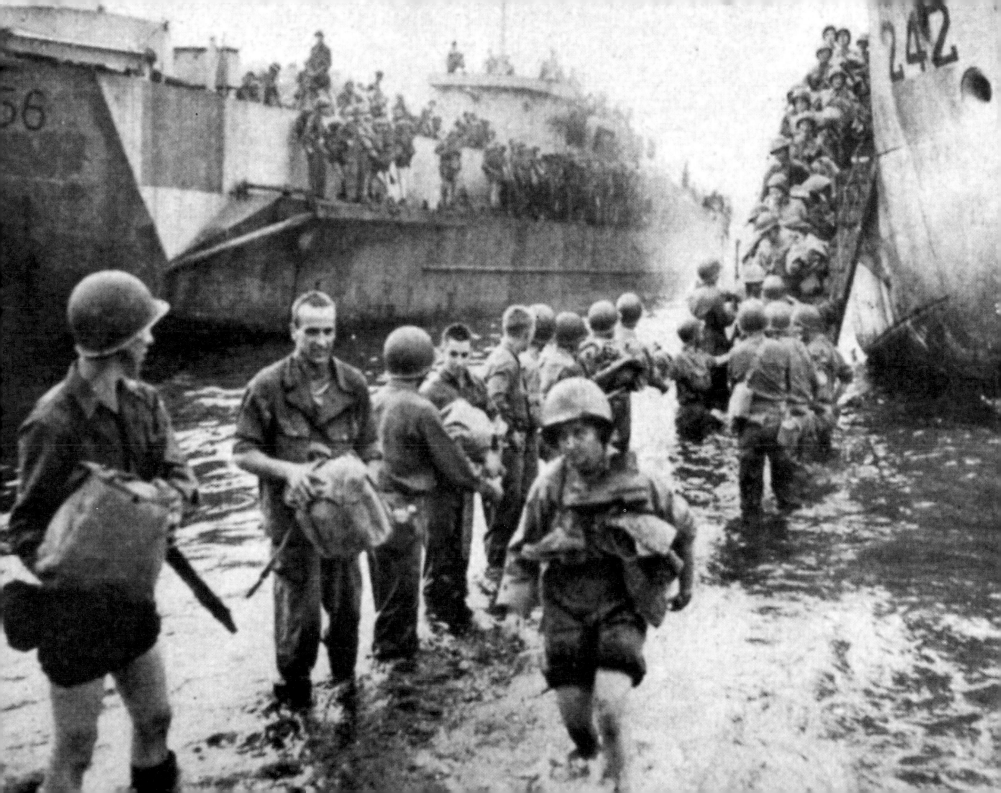

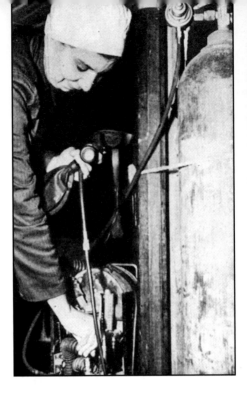

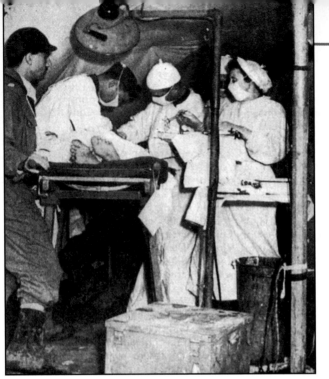

Army nurses in field hospitals in the European Theater of Operations. Left, a nurse anesthetist; right, a surgical scrub nurse.

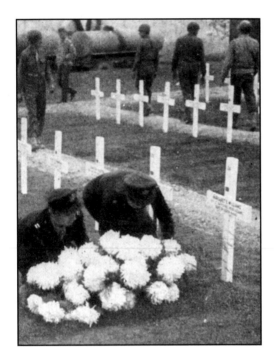

Decorating the grave of an Army nurse buried in a military cemetery in North Africa.

Kathleen R. Dial (St. Thomas, Memphis, Tenn.) was awarded the Distinguished Flying Cross, Air Medal, and Purple Heart. Reported to be the first woman to be awarded the Distinguished Flying Cross, she was caring for eighteen patients from the up-front lines in Guinea when the plane was forced to make a crash landing. Although she received fractures of the right shoulder, a dislocated hip, and a slight brain concussion, she directed the removal of the patients off the plane before she collapsed.

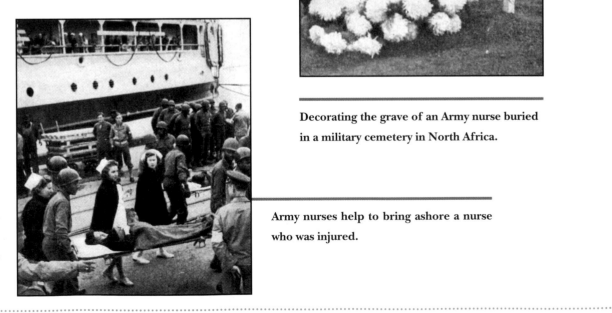

Army nurses help to bring ashore a nurse who was injured.

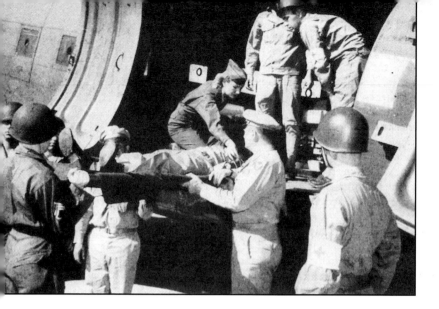

An air evacuation team in action.

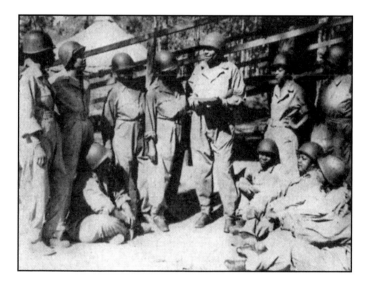

Negro nurses still served in segregated units during World War II. This unit was stationed in the southwest Pacific.

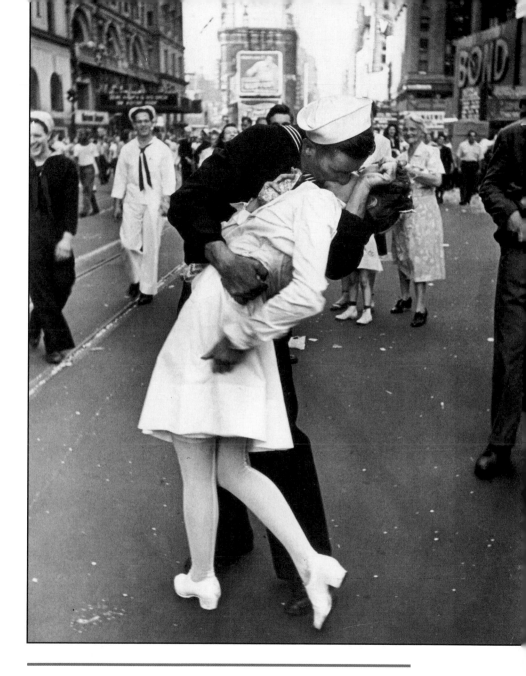

VJ Day in Times Square. Famous Alfred Eisenstadt photo of sailor kissing nurse.

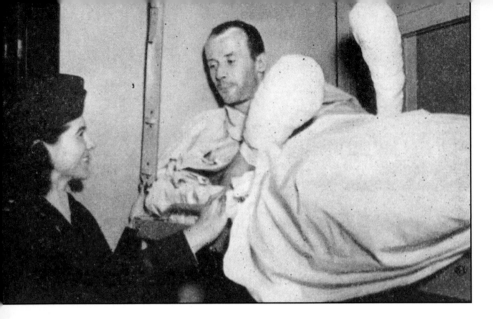

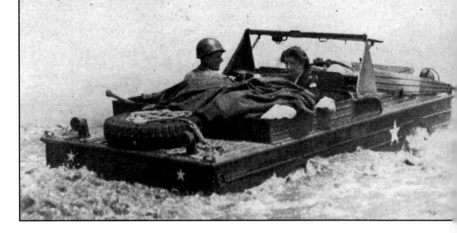

During the 1943 midwestern floods, a patient with acute appendicitis was transported by amphibian jeep across fifteen miles of swirling Arkansas River waters to a hospital.

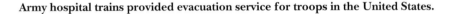

Army hospital trains provided evacuation service for troops in the United States.

"Trailer towns" —housing furnished by industry to secure workers during wartime—also had public health nursing centers and schools for the residents.

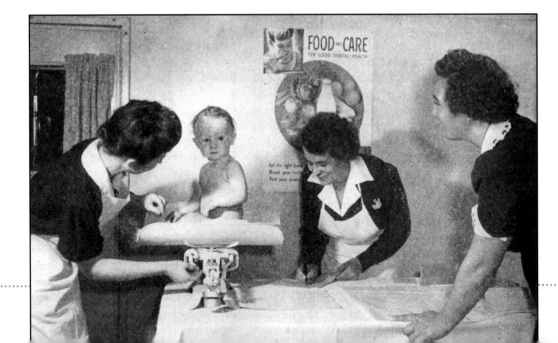

"To all nurses everywhere I would say: 'The people of America have no words with which to express their appreciation of your courage, your steadfastness, your faith. Wherever you serve, with the forces, or on the home front that needs you so sorely, too, know that our grateful hearts are with you. And may the infinite and eternal God constantly recharge you with His energy, His gentleness, His fortitude, and His divine love, that you may be upheld and strengthened in the work you have chosen to do. And may He give us all courage to uphold decency and honor and truth, until in His own time we come again to peace.'"

THE HONORABLE FRANCES PAYNE BOLTON
SEPTEMBER 1943

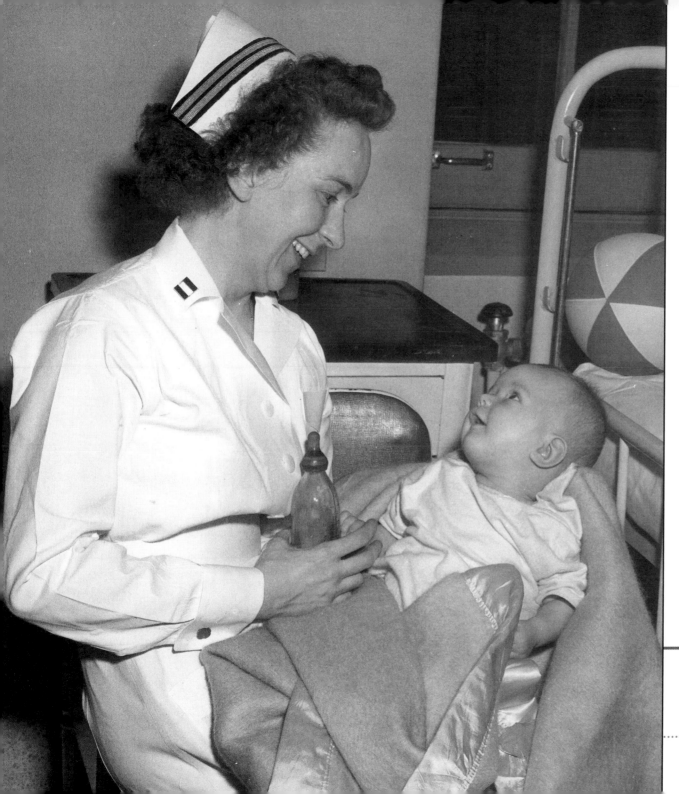

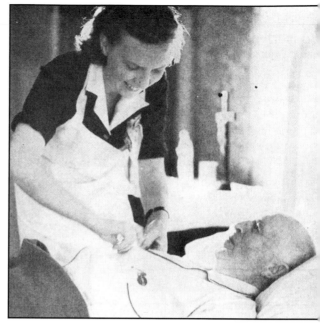

In almost every rooming house there is some lonely, elderly person whose life is brightened by the community nurse's visit.

After the war, some nurses returned home to continue where they left off.

One of the United Nations Relief and Rehabilitation Administration's camps in the Middle East, where more than 23,000 Yugoslav refugees were cared for.

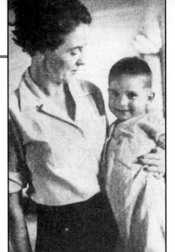

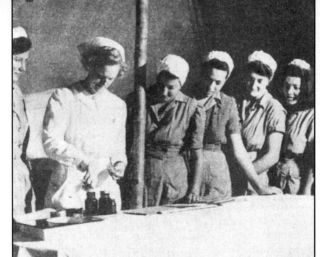

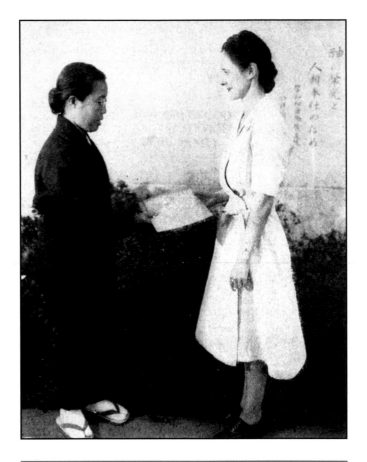

The end of the war meant the beginning of a new experience for nurses of the 42nd General Hospital, the first American medical unit to enter Japan. Here, the Japanese chief nurse turns over the keys of St. Luke's International Medical Center in Tokyo to Lt. Colonel Grace Dick, ANC, Chief Nurse of the 42nd General Hospital.

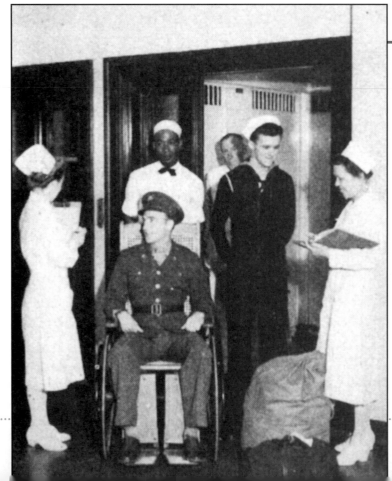

Thousands of World War II veterans, young men of military age, entered Veterans Administration hospitals for treatment and nursing care. There were female patients too—Army and Navy nurses, WAVES, WACS, SPARS, and Marine Corps women.

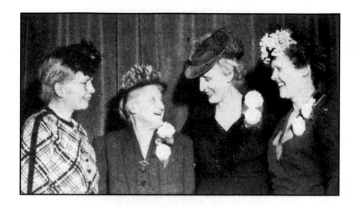

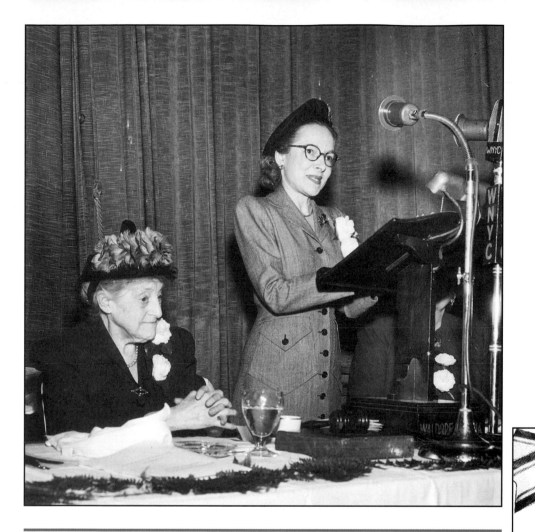

Actress Helen Hayes, speaking as the "average American," pays tribute to Annie Goodrich on her 80th birthday.

At the birthday celebration, Miss Goodrich and the presidents: (left) Marion Sheahan, President, National Organization for Public Health Nursing; at Miss Goodrich's left, Katharine J. Densford, President, American Nurses' Association; (right) Ruth Sleeper, President, National League of Nursing Education. Miss Goodrich was president of two of these national nursing organizations (the NLNE in 1906 and the ANA in 1915–1918) and was the first president of the Association of Collegiate Schools of Nursing.

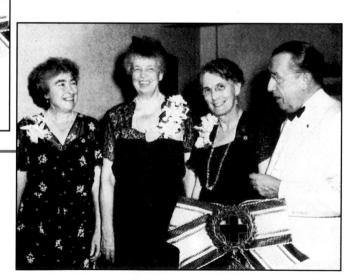

Congratulations were in order at the American National Red Cross Convention in 1949 to winners of the Florence Nightingale Award. Left to right: Alta Dines, award winner; Eleanor Roosevelt, award winner; Mary Roberts, AJN editor; and Basil O'Connor, president of the American Red Cross.

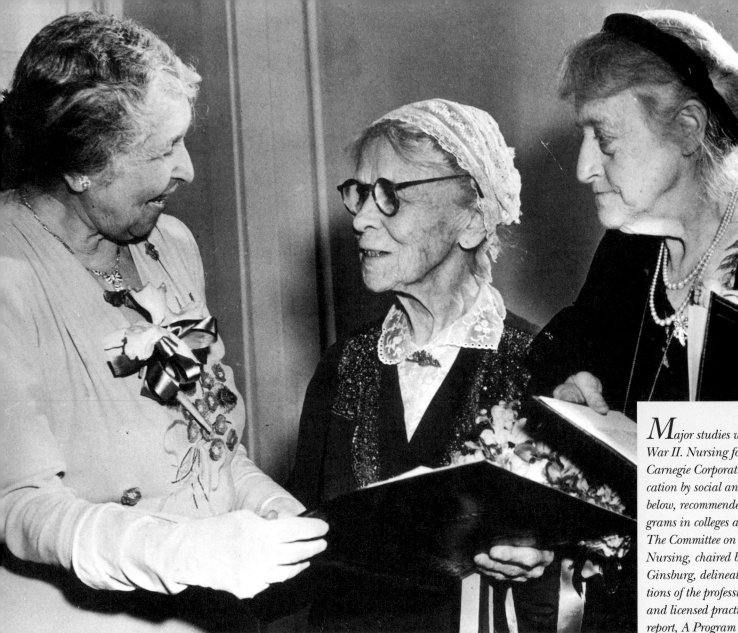

Left to right: Effie Taylor, Lavinia Dock, and Annie Goodrich at the International Council of Nurses meeting in Atlantic City, 1947.

Major studies were carried out following World War II. Nursing for the Future, the report of a Carnegie Corporation-sponsored study of nursing education by social anthropologist Esther Lucille Brown, below, recommended the development of nursing programs in colleges and universities. The Committee on the Function of Nursing, chaired by economist Eli Ginsburg, delineated the functions of the professional nurse and licensed practical nurse. The report, A Program for the Nursing Profession, predicted the development of "professional" and "semiprofessional" nurses.

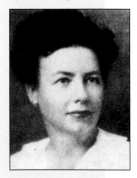

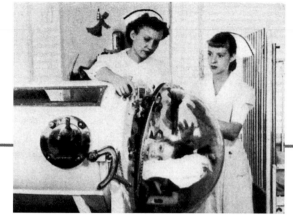

Laying the Groundwork for Change

1950–1959

The Fifties—some called them fabulous, others thought they were frightening. Civil defense was paramount, as people constantly worried about the threat of atomic warfare. And war did start—in 1950 in Korea—and Army and Navy nurses went there to serve in Mobile Army Surgical Hospital [MASH] units in hospitals, in Japan and the Philippines, on Navy ships and Air Force transport planes. The need for nurses would remain a critical problem throughout this decade.

At home, debates were flaring over nursing education—where, why, and how should a nurse be educated? In the traditional diploma school? In a baccalaureate program? With credit for previous courses, even those not taken in a university setting? And what about the value of experience? Out of research on the possibility of shortening three-year programs, the associate degree programs emerged and their numbers escalated, making them a voice to be listened to in the continuing debate.

Six nursing organizations merged into two in 1952—only the American Association of Industrial Nurses chose to go it alone. The new National League for Nursing set about realizing its charge—bringing professional and lay talents together to focus on nursing education, service, and public health.

The American Nurses Association was putting resources and energy into functions studies—determining what nurses were doing and what they should be doing. Concerns about economic security and the use of collective bargaining sparked interest in state associations and the development of local units in hospitals and public health agencies.

The expansion of hospitals under the Hill-Burton Act, the spread of voluntary health insurance, plus the demands of the military intensified the mounting demands for nursing personnel. Congress responded by passing the Health Amendments Act of 1956, setting up financial aid for federal traineeships that markedly affected nursing progress and would for decades to come.

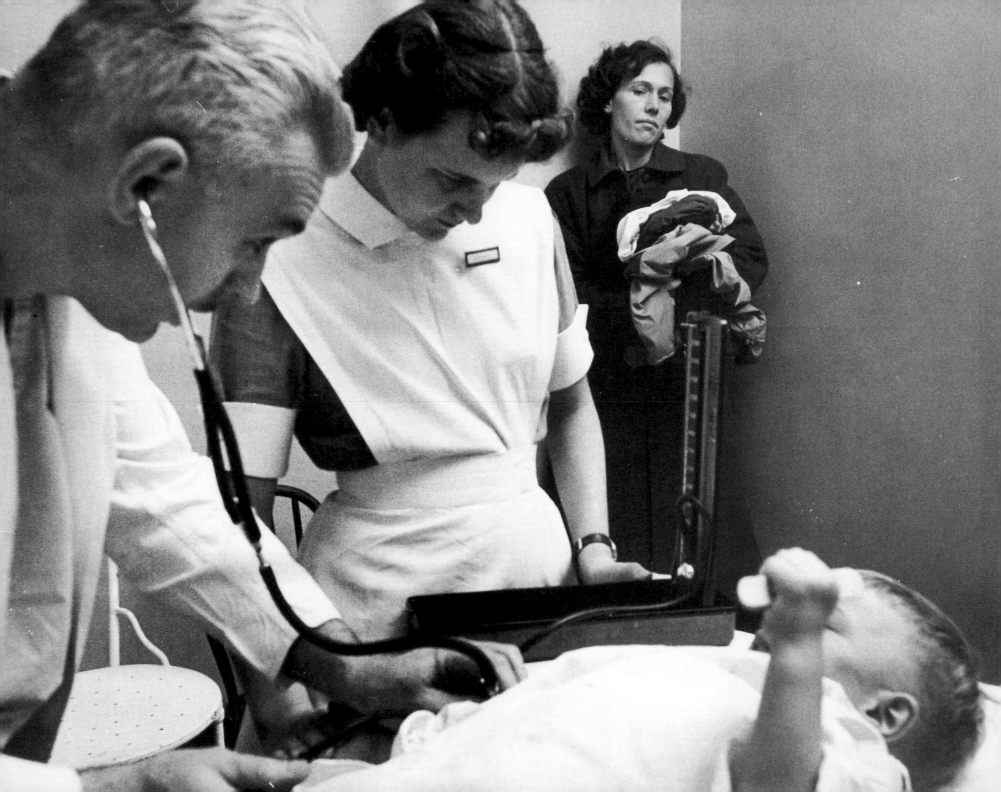

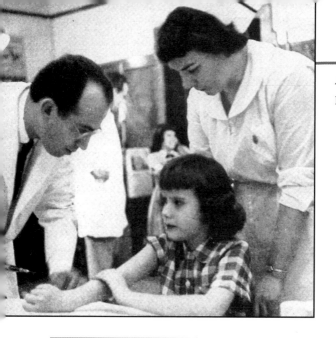

Administration of a new oral polio vaccine gets under way in a test at the University of Minnesota housing village. The new oral vaccine is available in capsule form, too.

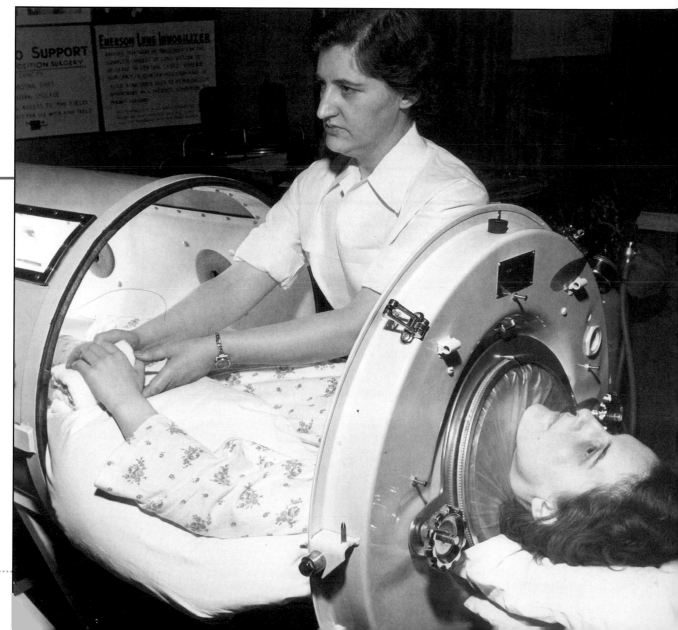

Poliomyelitis, the scourge known as infantile paralysis because its victims were most often children and young adults, caused pain, muscle spasm, bulbar and respiratory distress, and in many cases crippling paralysis.

Outbreaks crisscrossed the country and nurses recruited by the American Red Cross were flown to the hardest hit cities, with their expenses underwritten by the National Foundation for Infantile Paralysis.

Patients with respiratory paralysis were immobilized in Drinker respirators and required constant, relentless nursing care.

For patients with muscle spasm and persistent pain, hot packs were applied almost continuously for two weeks or until the pain abated and evaluation could determine the need for further treatment—intensive physical therapy, braces, surgery. In the mid-fifties, the miracle occurred—the development of a vaccine by Jonas Salk.

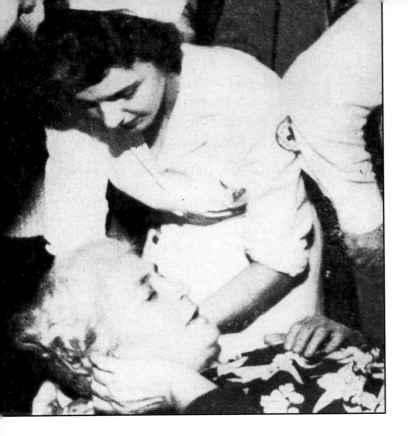

The *Fabulous* Fifties?

"*D*ecade of disasters" is what the Red Cross calls the fifties, known in other circles as fabulous.

Among the major disaster operations were those during the 1951 floods in Kansas, Missouri, Oklahoma, and Iowa; the eastern states floods of 1955; the western states floods of the same year. Then there were the operations that followed the collision and sinking of the Andrea Doria in 1956, hurricane Audrey of 1957, the mideastern states floods of January 1959.

"By almost any kind of arithmetic," the ARC booklet reports, "the fifties came out the worst decade our nation has ever known."

SEPTEMBER 1957

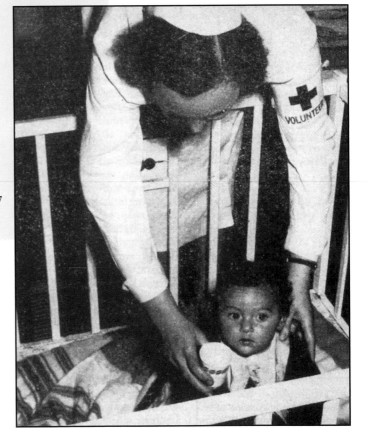

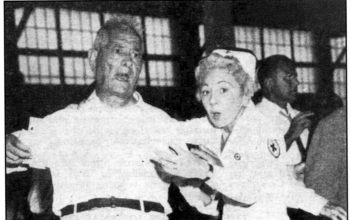

Taking a Stand on Health Insurance for the Aged

> *A Resolution on Health Insurance for Disabled, Retired, and Aged*
>
> *WHEREAS, necessary health services should be available to all people in this country without regard to their ability to purchase, and . . .*
>
> *WHEREAS, certain groups in our population, particularly the disabled, retired, and aged, are neither eligible nor able to avail themselves of voluntary health insurance, be it therefore*
>
> *RESOLVED, That the American Nurses Association supports the extension and improvement of the contributory social insurance to include health insurance for beneficiaries of old age, survivors, and disability insurance; and be it further*
>
> *RESOLVED, That nursing services, including nursing care in the home, be included as a benefit of any prepaid health insurance program.*

"The ANA's support of the principle of extending social security benefits to include health care is dramatic evidence of the independent thinking of which nursing is capable. Whether or not people agree with the position the ANA has taken, its willingness to stand up and be counted on a health issue facing the entire nation is a measure of nursing's courage, its maturity, and its professionalism."

EDITORIAL, SEPTEMBER 1958

The Journal also published, at the American Medical Association's request, an article explaining the AMA's opposition to the Forand health insurance bill:

"The group opposed to this concept—the American Medical Association, American Hospital Association, American Dental Association, American Nursing Home Association, U.S. Chamber of Commerce, American Farm Bureau Federation, the Blue Cross-Blue Shield, and the private health insurance industry, among many others—places its faith in traditional voluntary enterprise and resists government intervention. . . ."

SEPTEMBER 1958

The Forand bill failed and it was not until 1965 that health insurance for the aged (Medicare) would finally be established.

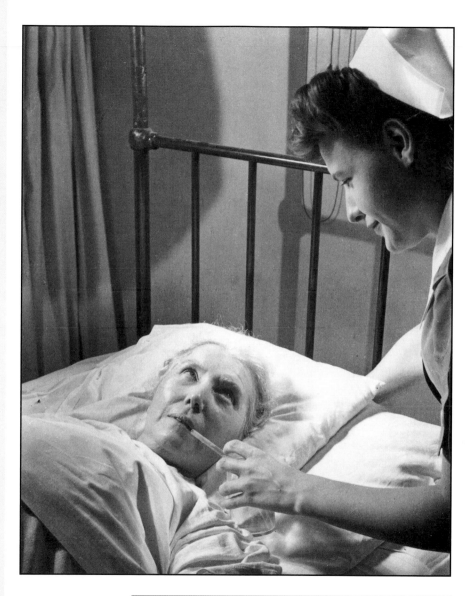

While the setting varies and specific tasks change, two indispensable components remain—the patient and the nurse, one needing, the other giving.

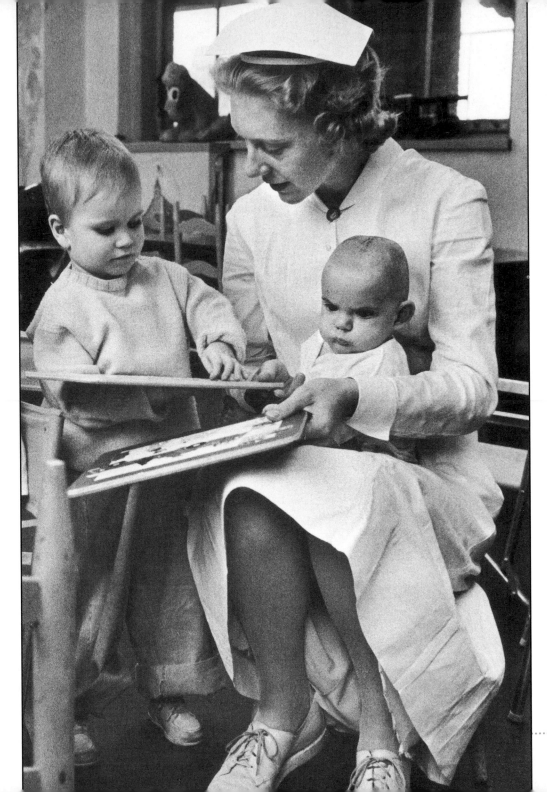

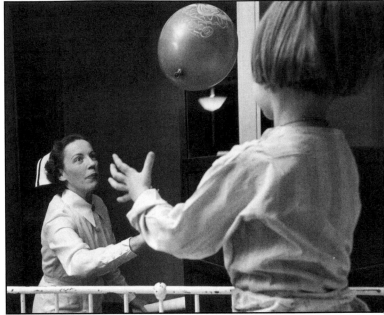

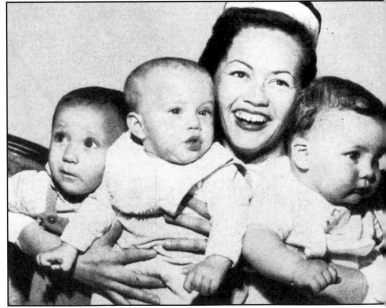

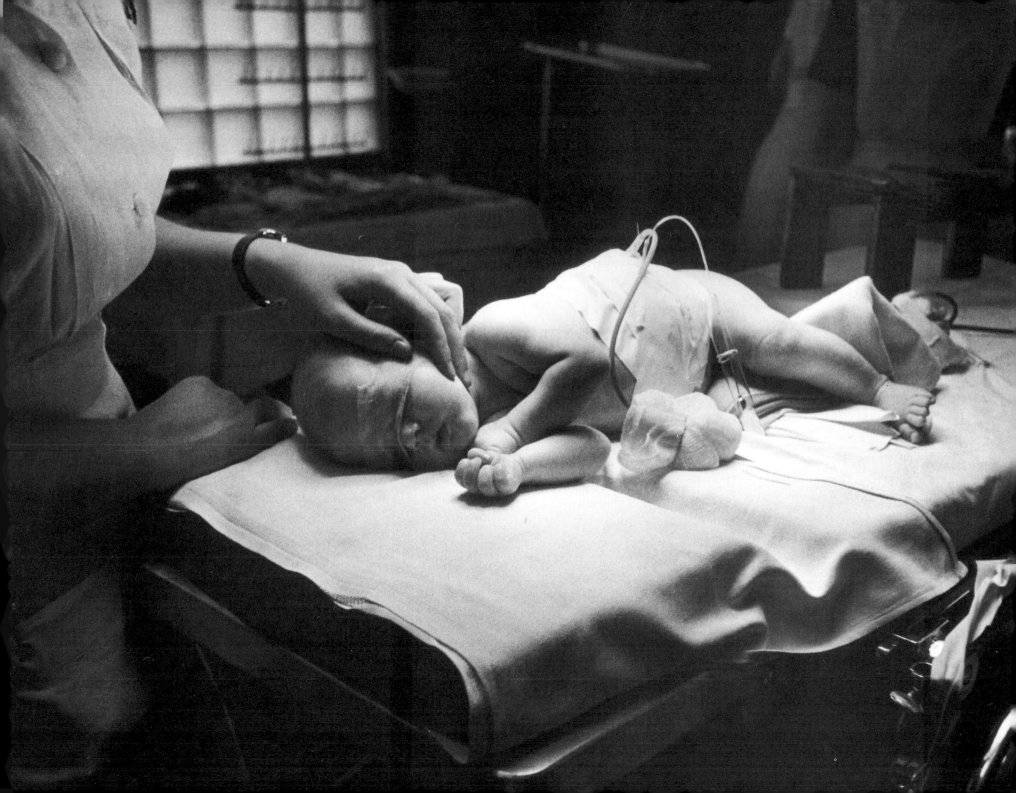

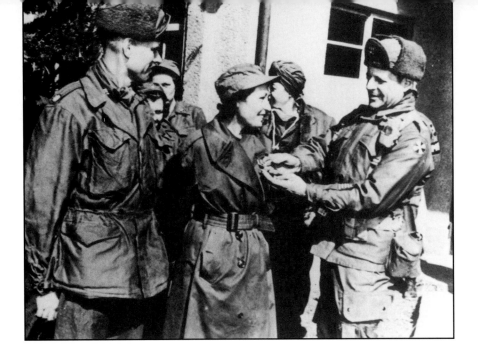

MASH units made their debut in the Korean War. Here, Lt. General Matthew Ridgway decorates Major Eunice Coleman, Chief Nurse, First Mobile Army Surgical Hospital, Korea.

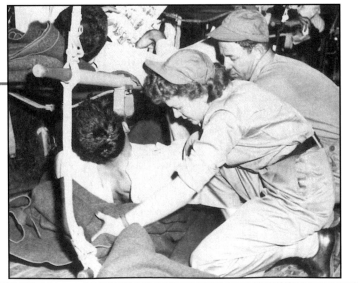

Flight nurse cares for an injured soldier in shock.

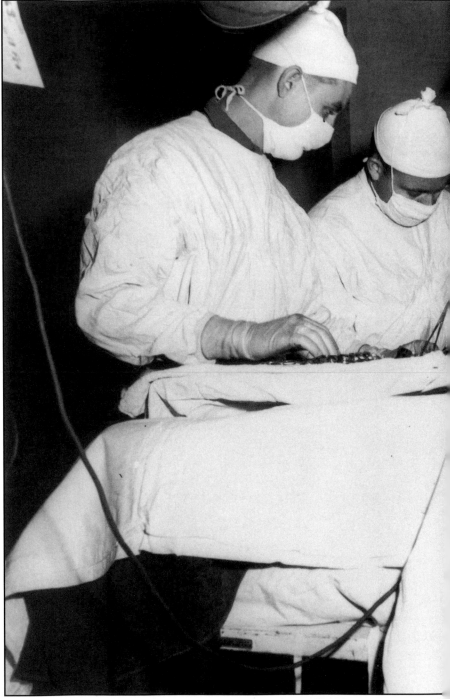

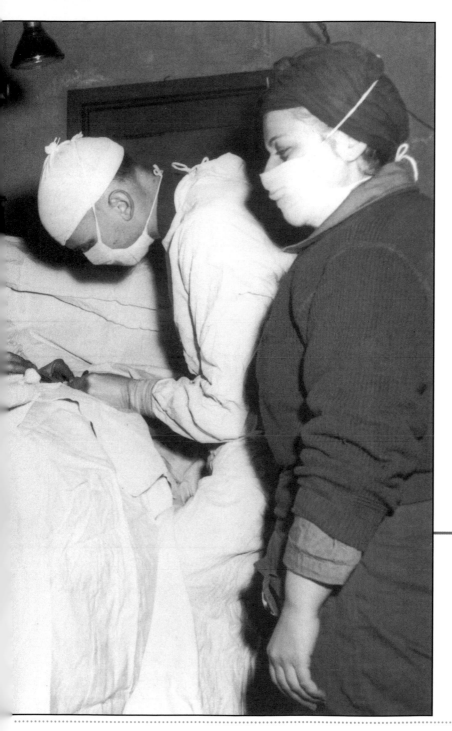

Surgery in a MASH unit.

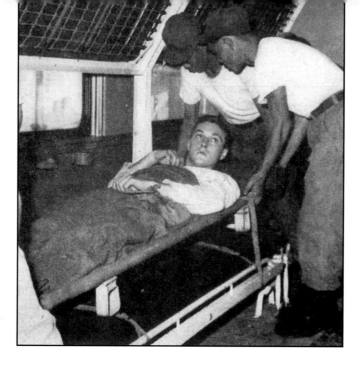

Hospital trains in Korea.

"Someone has said that if we all spoke the same language there would be no more war, and therefore we can suppose, no more chaos, no more crises. . . . But as nurses we have a common language. It is the language of a common purpose, and of sympathy and of understanding, and we do not necessarily have to express ourselves in words to know that our motives will be understood."

DAISY C. BRIDGES, Executive Secretary, International Council of Nurses

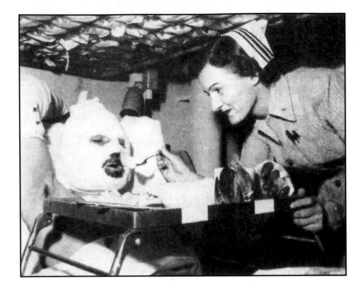

A little help with Thanksgiving dinner doesn't come amiss.

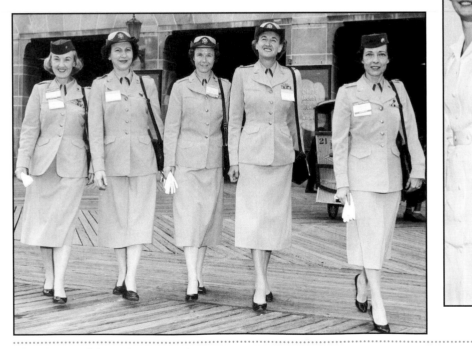

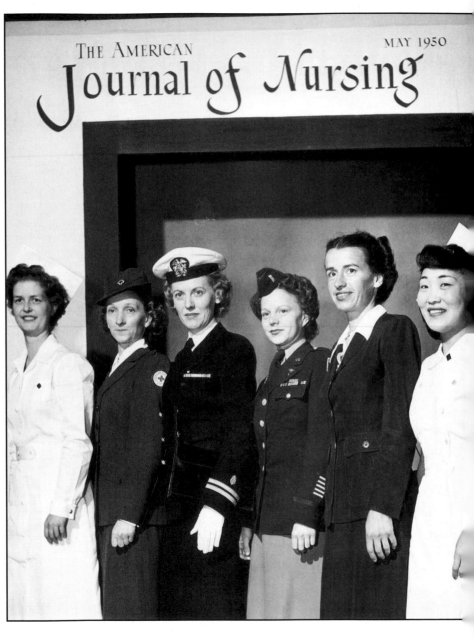

THE AMERICAN

Journal of Nursing

MAY 1950

Navy nurse and patient on board the USS *Haven* in Inchon Harbor, Korea.

*T*he good nurse says, *"I want to take care of you, and I know how to take care of you. You are safe with me."*

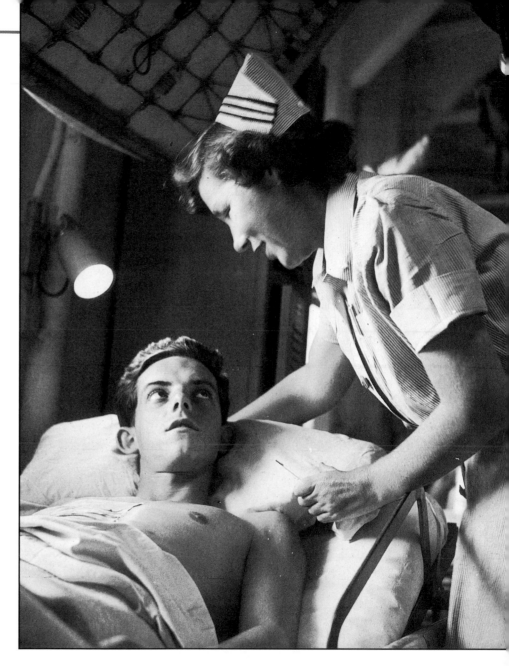

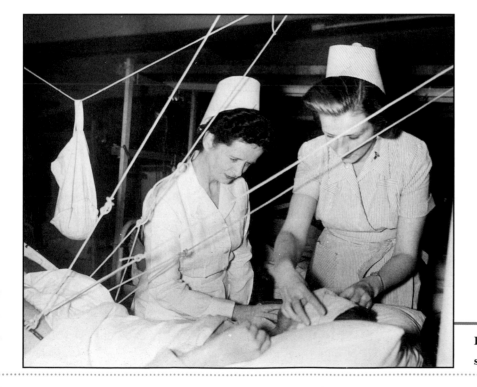

Following initial treatment at a MASH unit, many soldiers were then shipped to the Army hospital in Tokyo.

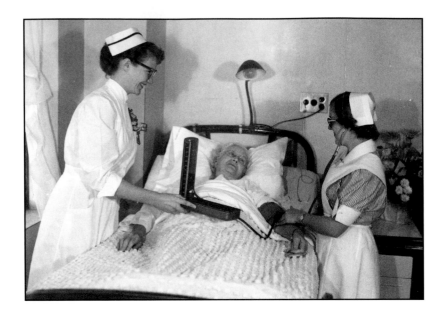

Nursing student learning basic skills.

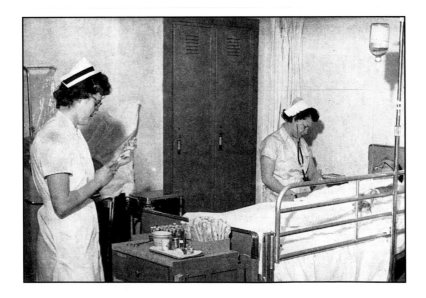

Early ICU, Manchester Memorial Hospital, Manchester, Connecticut.

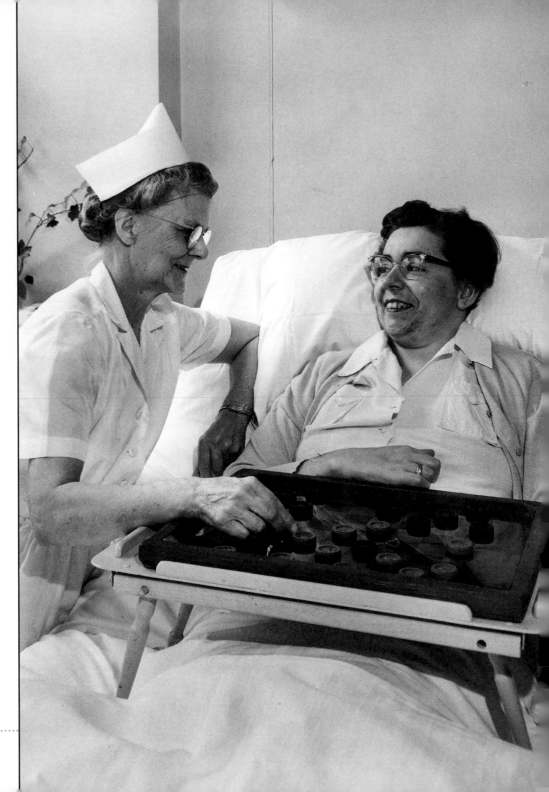

Commentary

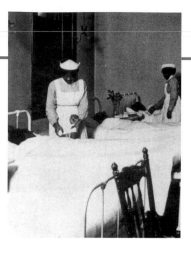

M. Elizabeth Carnegie

Human Rights

By 1896, many states, especially but not exclusively in the South, enacted statutes designed to separate the races in all aspects of life. Hospitals and nursing schools followed this pattern of segregation and discrimination in both the selection of students and the care of patients. It was this exclusion that forced the establishment of all-black hospitals and schools of nursing.

Because of discrimination, as early as 1900, black nurses in cities such as Norfolk, Washington, New York, and Chicago organized themselves into local clubs. And, in 1908, black nurses from all over the country came together in New York City to organize a national association. Known as the National Association of Colored Graduate Nurses (NACGN), the organization elected Martha Franklin, a graduate of Woman's Hospital in Philadelphia, as its president.

When the ANA was founded in 1896, membership was through the alumnae associations. When the states became the membership units of the ANA and membership was denied black nurses in southern states and the District of Columbia in 1916, the NACGN became the fighting force for the integration of black nurses into the organization. In 1961, Georgia was the last state to admit blacks to membership.

Despite their honorable service in the Spanish-American War in 1898, there were no black nurses among members of the Army Nurse Corps when it was formally established in 1901. And, regardless of the efforts of the NACGN and others, those black nurses who had volunteered their service during World War I were not accepted by the Army Nurse Corps until after the armistice had been signed in 1918. Only 18 were admitted, and their acceptance was likely due to the great need for nurses during the influenza pandemic.

At the time of Pearl Harbor in 1941, the NACGN was in the midst of a vigorous campaign to break down racial barriers in the Army and the Navy. Despite the Surgeon General's plea for nurses to enlist in the Armed Services, the Army had established a quota of 56 black nurses, and the Navy had flatly refused to admit any. Through the efforts of the NACGN, the Army quota was abolished before the end of the war, and the Navy dropped its color bar in January 1945. By the end of the war, over 500 black nurses had served in the Army and four in the Navy.

In 1946, the ANA launched a campaign to encourage all state and local associations to drop racial barriers to membership. In 1948, a policy was adopted that meetings be held only in integrated facilities. A special category of direct membership for black nurses in those states practicing discrimination was also created. This meant that black nurses in the South could bypass the states and join the ANA directly. It was also in 1948 that Estelle Massey Osborne became the first black nurse elected to the ANA Board of Directors.

On May 17, 1954, in the case of *Brown v. Board of Education of Topeka,* the Supreme Court unanimously reversed *Plessy v. Ferguson,* which had legalized segregation in 1896. On the basis of the fourteenth amendment, the court outlawed racial discrimination in public schools. With integration permitting black students to be admitted to formerly all-white schools, good black schools had difficulty attracting the number of qualified students who might otherwise have applied. Hence, a large number of these institutions closed.

Although the ANA bylaws for many years included a nondiscriminatory principle, in 1962 this was more appropriately placed within the statement of purposes of the organization. This platform states that the Association will "encourage all members, unrestricted by consideration of nationality, race, creed, or color, to participate fully in association activities and to work for full access to employment and educational opportunities for nursing."

At the 1970 ANA convention, however, black nurse members voiced their concern over a number of issues, including the absence of black nurses

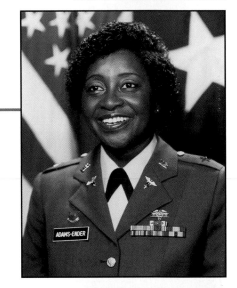

Mary E. P. Mahoney, first black professional nurse.

Brigadier General Clara Adams-Ender, Army Nurse Corps.

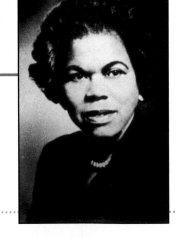

Estelle Osborne, first black nurse elected to ANA Board of Directors.

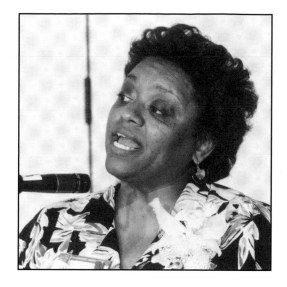

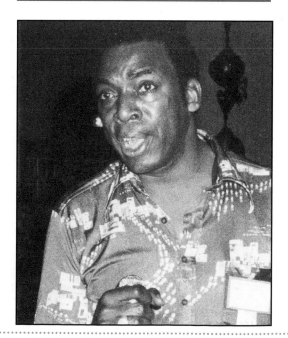

Above, Barbara Nichols, first black president, ANA. Below, Charles Hargett, New York delegate to the 1978 ANA Convention.

in leadership positions in the organization; limited opportunities for blacks to share in shaping ANA policies and priorities; limited recognition of the black nurse's contribution to nursing; no significant increases in the number of black registered nurses; and persistent tokenism.

At the 1972 convention, the ANA passed an affirmative action resolution calling for a task force to develop and implement a program to correct inequities. At the same convention, the House of Delegates adopted a comprehensive resolution on the Universal Declaration of Human Rights. This placed the organization on record in support of specific human rights and race relations issues. For example, the ANA now took a formal stand on fair employment opportunities, equal access to education, and implementation of the 1965 Civil Rights Act.

An Affirmative Action Task Force was established in 1972, and, in 1976, a Commission (later retitled Cabinet) on Human Rights. Under the jurisdiction of this Cabinet was a Council on Intercultural Nursing, which was set up to improve the quality of nursing care by being responsive to cultural and ethnic variances among consumers and to promote the inclusion of cultural diversity in the curriculum of nursing programs. In 1984, the Council on Intercultural Nursing was renamed the Council on Cultural Diversity in Nursing Practice. Its new purpose was to improve nursing practice based on the inclusion of cultural conditions, values, beliefs, and attitudes.

In 1978, for the first time in the history of the ANA, Barbara Nichols, a black nurse, was elected president. At the 1980 convention, she was voted to a second two-year term. In 1996, the ANA elected its second black president, Beverly Malone, who was reelected in 1998.

In 1982, following an extensive study, the ANA reorganized, disbanding its cabinets, including the Cabinet on Human Rights. The strands of ethics, human rights, nursing education, and nursing research were restructured as part of the work of all ANA units. In 1990, a Center for Ethics and Human Rights was established, charged with the responsibility of ensuring that ethics and human rights are considered in all activities of the ANA.

The late 1960s and early 1970s were characterized by the development of increasingly diverse health needs, which placed new demands on nursing. Changing attitudes and values within society and nursing created a movement to provide opportunities in the field to a broader segment of society. Recruitment efforts were directed toward particular minority groups, including disadvantaged youth, men, and others not previously encouraged to enter the field.

Established in 1973 under the aegis of the ANA, the American Academy of Nursing is composed of over 1,000 nursing leaders in practice, education, research, management, and policy-making. Among the 36 charter Fellows were two black nurses—Rhetaugh Dumas and Geraldene Felton— and three black women are also among the honorary Fellows—Estelle Massey Osborne, Marie Bourgeois, and Hattie Bessent. In addition, the Academy has elected three black presidents—M. Elizabeth Carnegie, Vernice Ferguson, and Rhetaugh Dumas.

One of the most successful ongoing ANA projects, established in 1974, is the Minority Fellowship Program, funded by the National Institute of Mental Health. The program was designed to increase the number of doctorally prepared ethnic/racial minority nurse researchers and to provide scientific data derived from research on ethnic/racial minority clientele as a basis for quality mental health and nursing service delivery. Over 200 minority nurses—blacks, Hispanics, Asians, and American Indians—have earned doctoral degrees through this program.

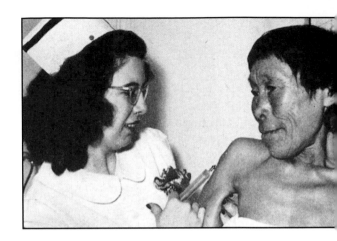

Public health nursing with the Indian Health Service in Alaska.

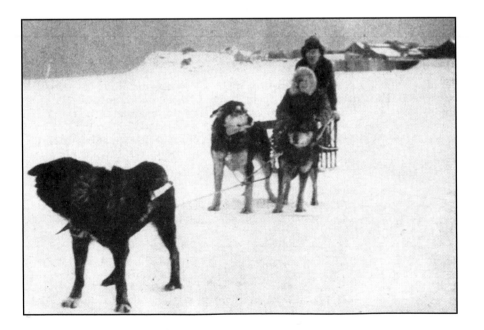

In Alaska, in the winter, the nurse may make her rounds by dog sled.

Public health nurse, North Carolina.

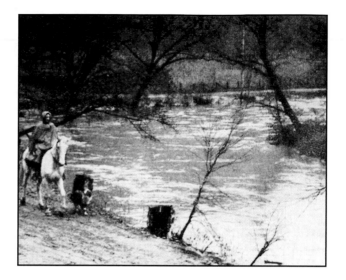

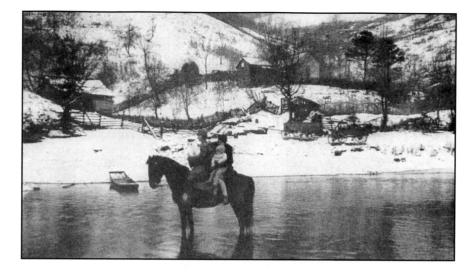

By the 1950s, the Frontier Nursing Service covered four Kentucky counties. Twelve nurse-midwives covered a 700-square-mile area and managed eight health care centers scattered across the counties.

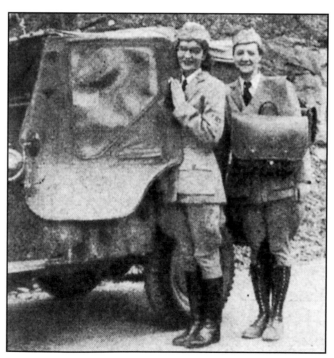

"America has made two unique contributions to medicine—the Panama Canal and the public health nurse."

WILLIAM WELCH, MD.

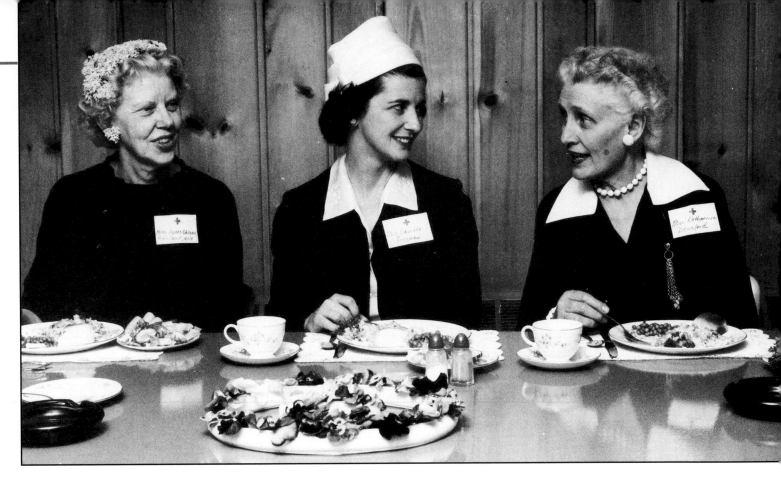

Enjoying a mid-meeting luncheon,
(left to right) Agnes Ohlson,
Mrs. Orville Freeman, wife of the
Minnesota governor, and
Katherine Densford.

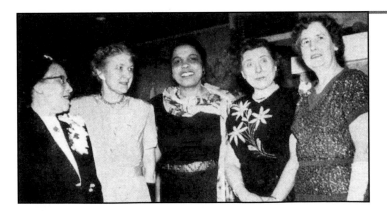

Five nursing presidents in 1951
(left to right): Mabel K. Staupers,
NACGN; Agnes Gelinas, NLNE;
Estelle M. Osborne, former president
of NACGN; Emilie G. Sargent,
NOPHN; Elizabeth K. Porter,
ANA.

A profession's beginnings, came a "little bit out of loneliness, finding someone else to talk with who knows the same things and does the same things." Next, these professional people begin to worry about "the members of their group who aren't as good as the others. . . . At that point they start talking about standards."

MARGARET MEAD
at the 1956 ANA Convention

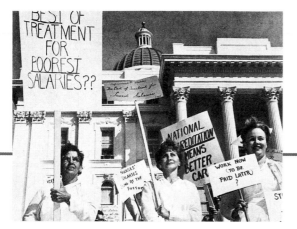

The Turbulent Sixties

1960–1969

The 1960s was a time of great social ferment—campuses in chaos; freedom marches; race riots; the horror of the assassinations of John Kennedy, Robert Kennedy, and Martin Luther King, Jr.; and the agony over the war in Vietnam.

But the 1960s also saw some remarkable advances in nursing and health care. For example, coronary care units—first tested in Hays, Kansas, then in Philadelphia and New York—were established in hospitals all over the country. The lives of hundreds of thousands of cardiac patients have since been saved because nurses monitored their ECGs and corrected dangerous irregular rhythms. The introduction of tranquilizers, oral contraceptives, polio vaccine, measles vaccine, L-dopa, semisynthetic penicillin, and new chemotherapy agents are other examples of major medical advances.

During this decade, demands for care also increased. In 1965, Medicare and Medicaid became law, making care available to the burgeoning over-65 population and to the poor. The spreading war in Vietnam heightened the needs of the military, and the nursing shortage in hospitals intensified. Again there was talk of a draft of nurses, but the common feeling was that this could occur only if there was a draft of all women.

The 1960s were also characterized by nurses becoming more proactive about their economic situation. The Bureau of Labor Statistics figures for 1963-1964 showed general duty nurses' salaries at $4,500. In comparison, teachers were averaging $6,325, and secretaries were making $5,170 a year. Nurses and the American Nurses Association (ANA) continued the fight to raise earnings. In 1968, the ANA's no-strike clause was rescinded.

In 1965, the ANA Board adopted the Position Paper on Education for Nursing, which called for baccalaureate education for future practitioners and proved to be explosive. Perhaps most controversial in the paper was the identification of "professional" nursing practice with baccalaureate education and the term "technical" nursing practice with diploma and associate degree education. The controversy continues to this day.

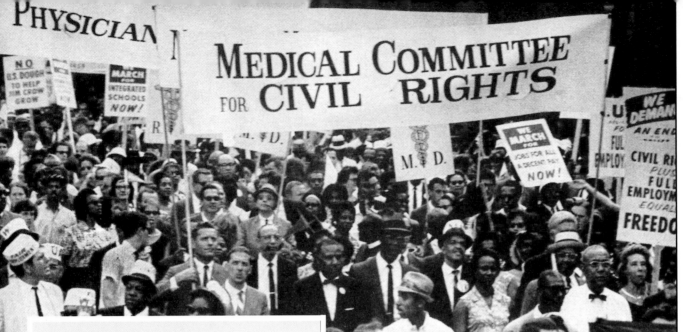

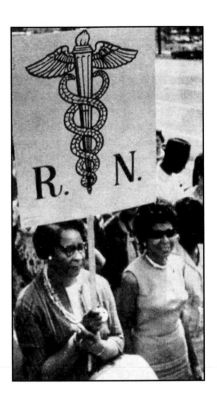

Civil Rights March on Washington, August 1963

In the historic August 28 March on Washington, nurses were seen demonstrating both their personal belief in the rights of all citizens, and their capacity to give skilled emergency care to the ill.

Some nurses marched with the Medical Committee for Civil Rights; others helped man the 25 first aid stations located along the lines of the march.

By 6:00 P.M. the vast sea of people which had demonstrated the best of humanity, both in intentions and performance, had gone. Still at their posts, however were the police who had smiled upon the marchers, and the nurses who had cared for them.

OCTOBER 1963

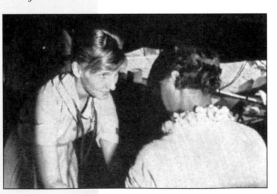

Under the Medical Committee for Civil Rights banner, nurses and other health care workers join the 200,000 marchers leaving the Washington Monument.

Ethel Underwood, public health nurse with New York's Community Service Society, and Rachel Robinson (Mrs. Jackie), psychiatric nursing supervisor, Albert Einstein College of Medicine.

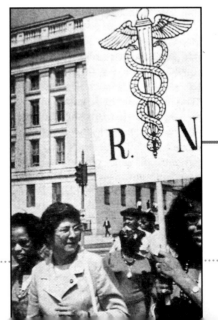

Ianthe Harris, ANA staff, Barbara Schutt, *AJN* editor, and Georgia Pollard, public health nurse, Community Service Society, march under another RN placard.

Nurses were everywhere with the Peace Corps—the Near East, the Far East, in Africa and South America. Over 400 nurses volunteered for service in 26 countries . . .

in Malaya . . .

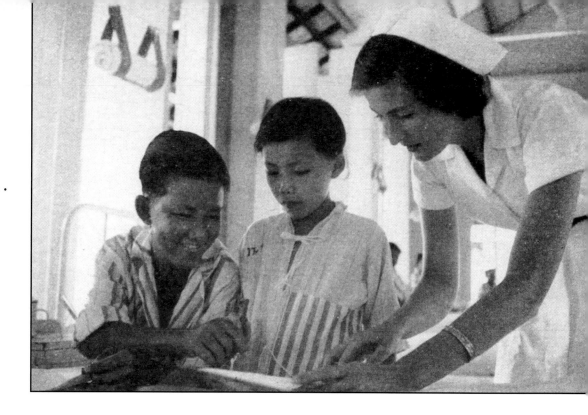

in Brazil . . .

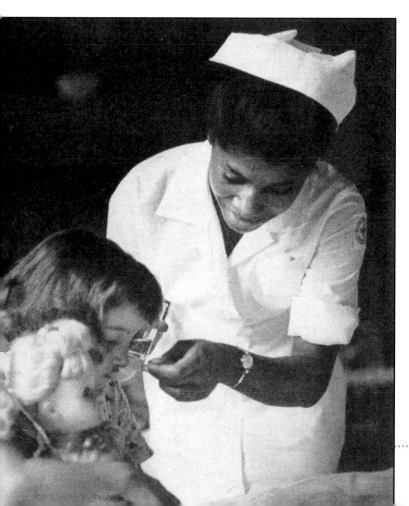

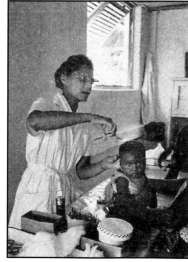

in Togo . . .   in Afghanistan . . .

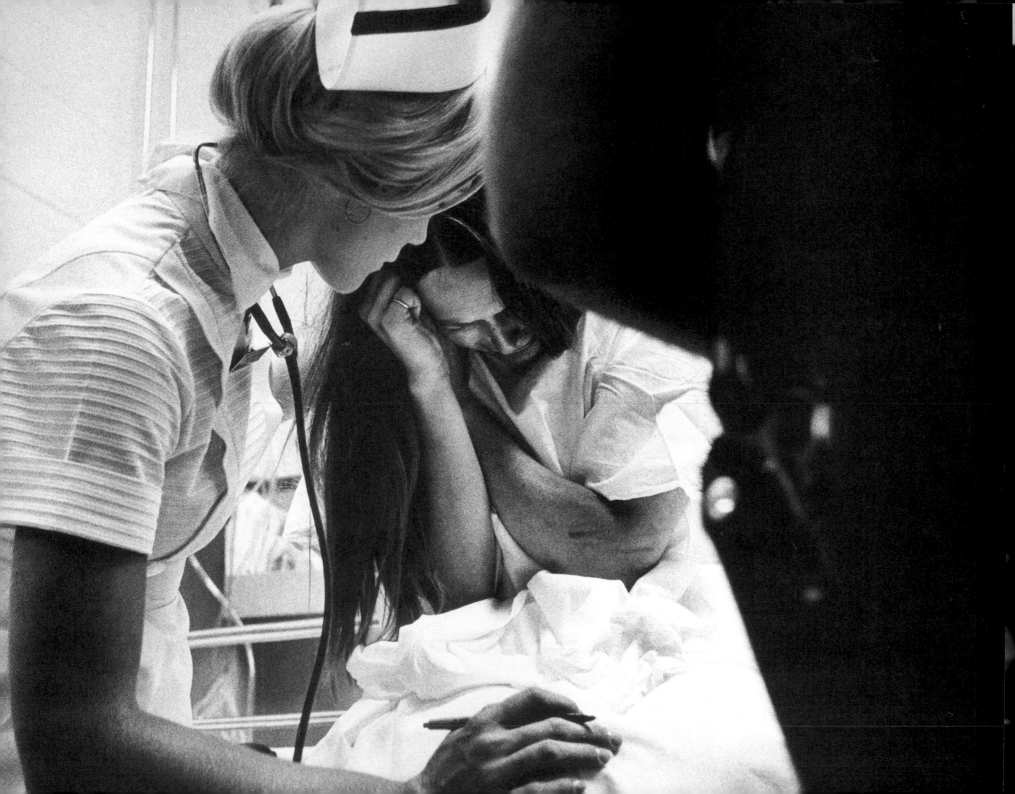

"It is no paradox that nursing has made some of its major strides during war. Nursing's means of participation in war has always been a waging of peace within it. Less important to many a soldier than the patching up of his injuries has been the very presence of the nurse who symbolized to him warmth and caring and hopefulness, bringing a murmur of peace within the sounds of war."

EDITORIAL, DECEMBER 1963

Army Nurse Corps Steps Up Recruitment in Support of General Military Build-Up

WASHINGTON, DC. The Army Nurse Corps is making an all-out effort to gain 500 professional nurses by the end of this year. This effort is made necessary by the current build-up in overall Army strength. The nurses are needed to fill expanded needs at training centers and to replace military nurses who are volunteering for service in Vietnam.

DECEMBER 1965

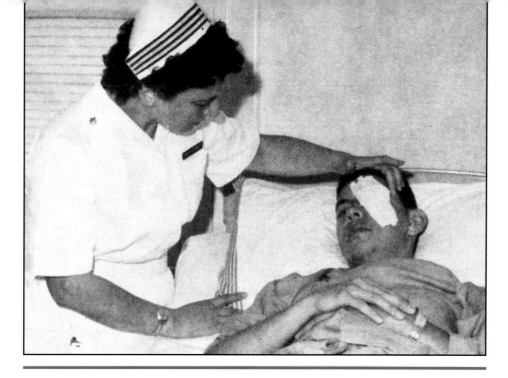

Navy nurse prepares patient to be airlifted home. He suffered eye injury during a Vietcong grenade attack.

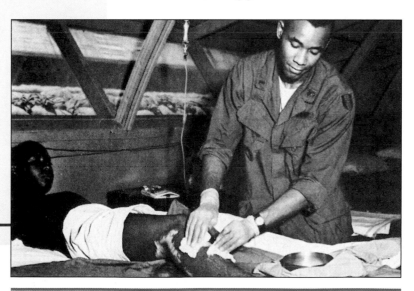

In contrast to previous wars, male nurses are highly visible in Vietnam.

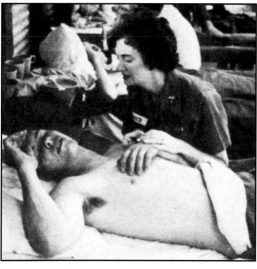

In Nha Trang field hospital, Army nurse tends to injured patient.

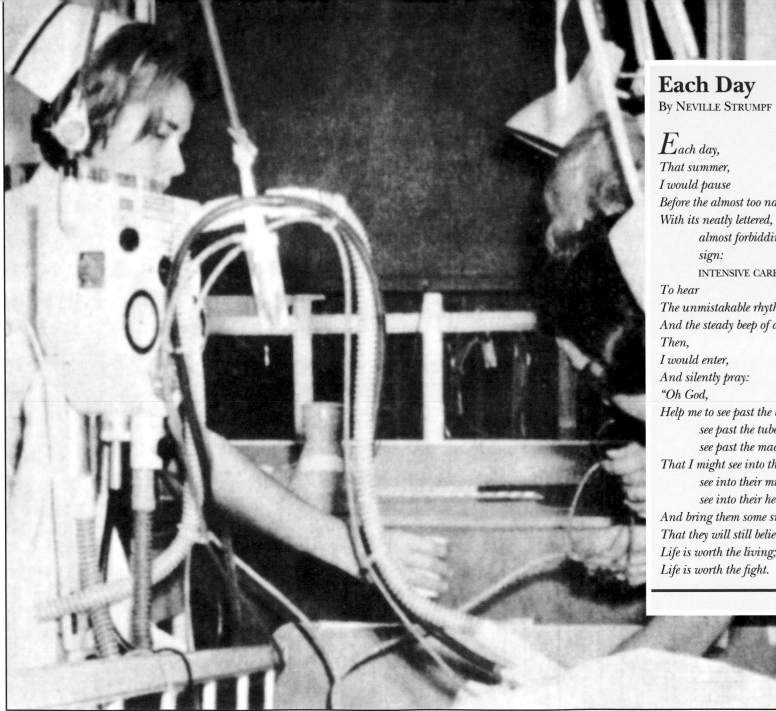

Each Day

By Neville Strumpf

Each day,
That summer,
I would pause
Before the almost too narrow door,
With its neatly lettered,
  almost forbidding,
  sign:
  INTENSIVE CARE UNIT
To hear
The unmistakable rhythmic gush of a respirator,
And the steady beep of a monitor.
Then,
I would enter,
And silently pray:
"Oh God,
Help me to see past the bottles,
  see past the tubes,
  see past the machines,
That I might see into their eyes,
  see into their minds,
  see into their hearts,
And bring them some small part of my healthy self,
That they will still believe
Life is worth the living;
Life is worth the fight.

Commentary

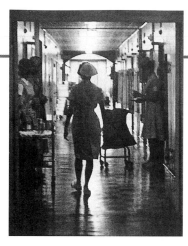

Luther Christman

The Interrelationship Between Nurses and Hospitals

In the early 1900s, most health care took place in the home under the direction of the family physician. Hospitals were a last resort, except for required or emergency surgical care. This pattern persisted during most of the first half of the century. During this time, much of the population was spread throughout small towns and rural settings. The growth of home health care organizations was blunted because financial support could not be mustered easily. With World War II, however, there was a sudden growth of large cities, as the United States became a dynamic manufacturing nation. The population shifted to manufacturing and commercial settings, where there was an amassing of health care facilities.

The Nightingale model of conjoint nursing service and education was introduced into this country when hospital nursing schools were first being established. The high marriage rate and subsequent dropout of nurses from the workforce, however, resulted in short careers. The practice of recruiting white women for the nursing vocation has historically deprived the profession of the talents of men and of minority women. Today, registered nurses remain 85 percent white and female.

The isolation of nurses in hospital schools of nursing had other negative effects. Nurses lacked the opportunity to explore academic and scientific concepts with students of differing backgrounds. In addition, the quality of instruction in the sciences was questionable; courses in hospital schools may not have been as rigorous as those taught in multidisciplinary higher education settings. Throughout their professional life, graduates of these schools tended to learn new concepts by a trickle effect from other disciplines in the workplace.

Another problem that nurses working in hospitals have historically faced is low wages. This condition is linked to the philosophy of Florence Nightingale, who held that nurses should draw satisfaction from being helpful, rather than from monetary compensation. Around the world, nurses have become mired at these low income levels. In 1947, nurses in the United States even lost the protection of the National Labor Relations Act (NLRA) when the Taft-Hartley law was enacted, and nonprofit hospitals were made exempt from compliance with NLRA tenets. This situation went unchanged until 1974.

For about the first half of this century, students as well as nursing staff typically worked ten hours a day for six days a week. Students worked both day and night shifts. Their work time included class hours, and what limited free time there was had to be used for study. Because of these conditions, only an extremely small percentage of graduates sought further education.

The Hill-Burton Act, passed after World War II to erect hospitals throughout the nation, had a negative effect on nursing. Its sponsors were highly motivated to increase the availability of health care, but they neglected to write a companion bill to fund the professionals needed to staff these new facilities adequately. As a result, nurses became much more removed from direct patient care and, instead, found themselves managing aides and other auxiliary staff. Because of these changes, the quality of patient care was in all likelihood compromised. As research indicates, although nurses aides are paid lower salaries, because of their limited skills they ultimately do not provide the best patient care or save hospitals money.

The interrelationship nurses have historically had with hospitals does not have to be so troubled. In fact, a powerfully educated nursing profession, because of its binding role with patients, has the potential to be a very dominant force within hospitals. Nurses could form a self-governing organization, similar to that of the medical staff. Strong patient satisfaction with nursing care would generate positive media attention and support, which in turn would award nurses increasing respect and concessions by the administrators in the health care system.

Nurses are everywhere . . .

on country roads . . .

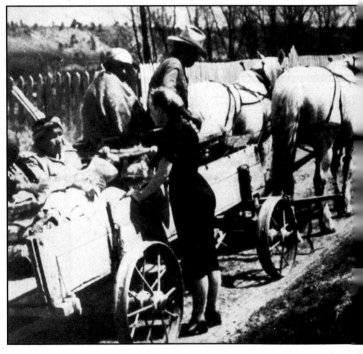

The public health nurse cares for her patients anywhere she can find them. It doesn't faze her a bit that many of the families she serves are almost continually on the move; she moves too.

on rooftops . . .

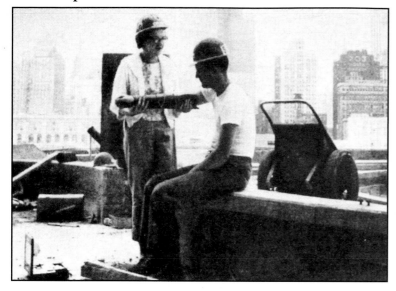

in hospitals . . .

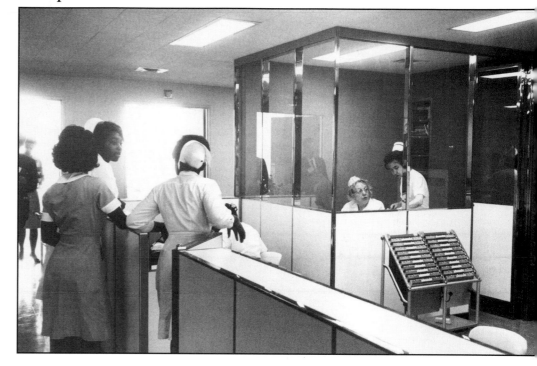

in Alaska . . .

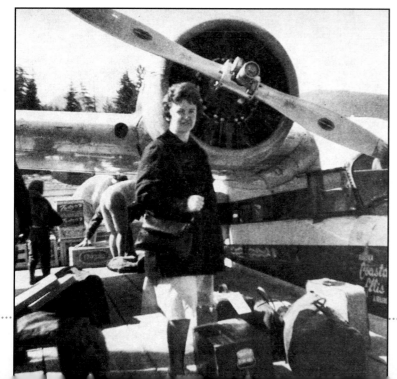

in the alleys of inner cities . . .

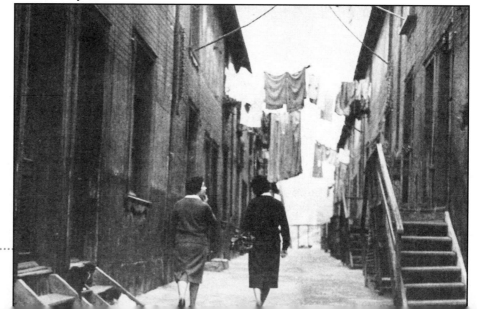

115

in mid-western schools . . .

in the rural South . . .

Nurses of District 3, Indiana State Nurses Association, Terre Haute, Indiana had a large part in getting a first dose of Sabin polio vaccine to 60,000 people in a community program.

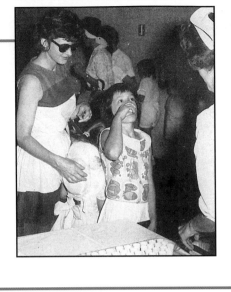

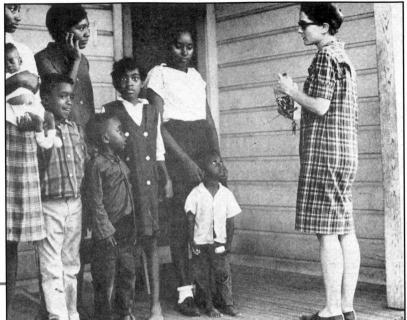

Holmes County, Mississippi—Nutrition teaching plays an important role in home visits.

in day care centers and clinics . . .

and on the west coast—

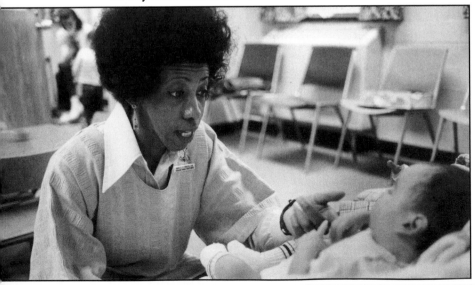

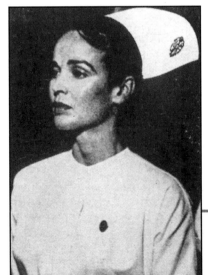

Kathryn Crosby, in private life Mrs. Bing Crosby, graduates from Queen of Angels School of Nursing, Los Angeles.

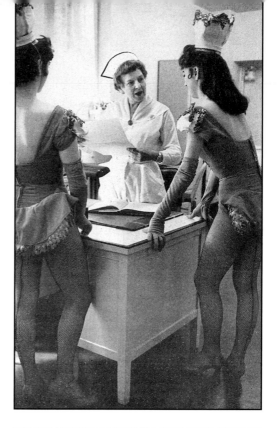

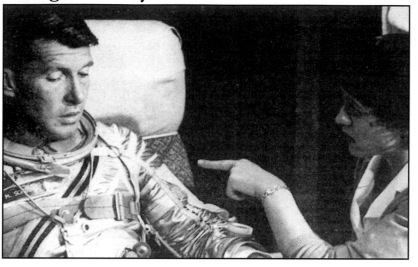

Cape Canaveral, Florida—Astronaut Walter Schirra discusses aspects of flight with his nurse.

New York City—Keeping the Rockettes in good shape at Radio City Music Hall.

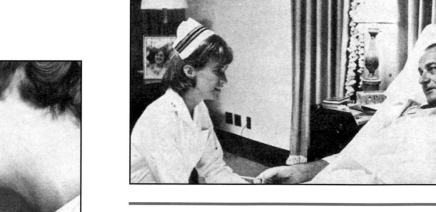

Washington, DC—This White House nurse "specialed" President Lyndon Johnson during his recent hospitalization for a cholecystectomy. A Navy nurse is regularly assigned to the White House.

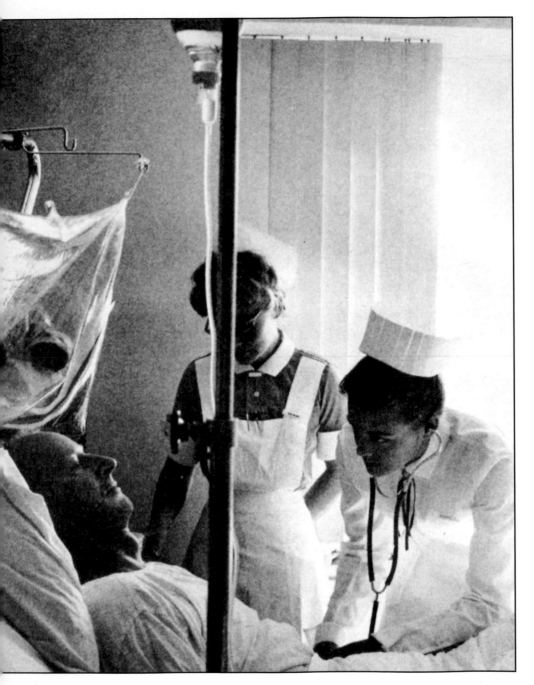

"*The care of the dying demands all that we can do to enable patients to live until they die. It includes the care of the family, the mind, and the spirit as well as the care of the body. All these are so interwoven that it is hard to consider them separately. I believe, however, that the most important factor of all is an atmosphere of such welcome and confidence that a patient can end her talk with me by saying, 'But it's so wonderful to begin to feel safe again.'*"

CICELY SAUNDERS, founder of the world-wide hospice movement

MARCH 1965

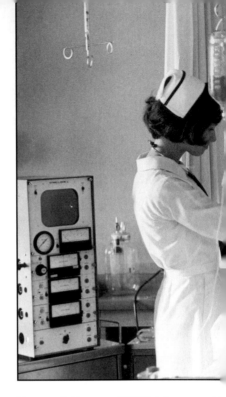

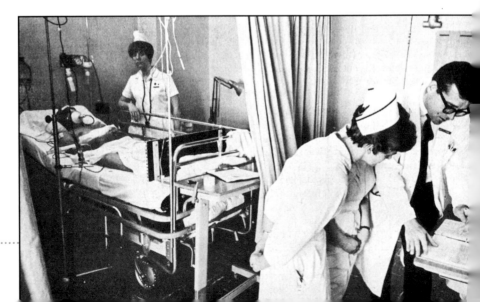

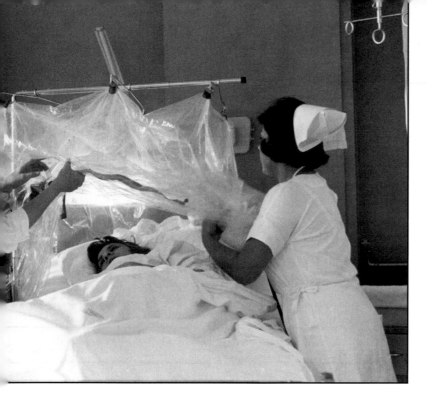

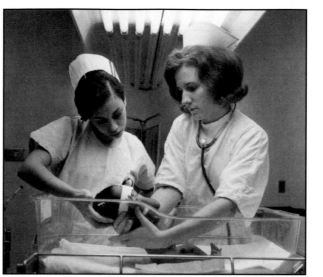

"*In our contacts with such elemental facts as suffering and death, we learn to disregard beauty, standing, intelligence, wit, and all those assets that people have. The dying have nothing; they tenuously are. And it is what they are that we fight to keep.*"

SISTER MADELEINE CLEMENCE
MARCH 1966

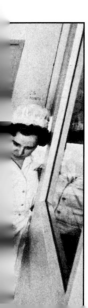

"*It is becoming increasingly apparent that the hospital of the not-too-distant future may be an enormous complex housing only patients requiring highly specialized medical and nursing care. It is envisioned by many that special care units will be large (30 beds or more) and that they will be exquisitely equipped and staffed. It may become economically feasible to hospitalize only the critically ill.*"

DONNA ZSCHOCHE
LILLIAN E. BROWN
NOVEMBER 1969

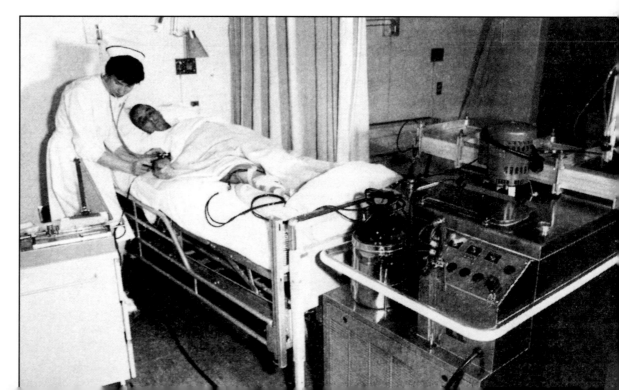

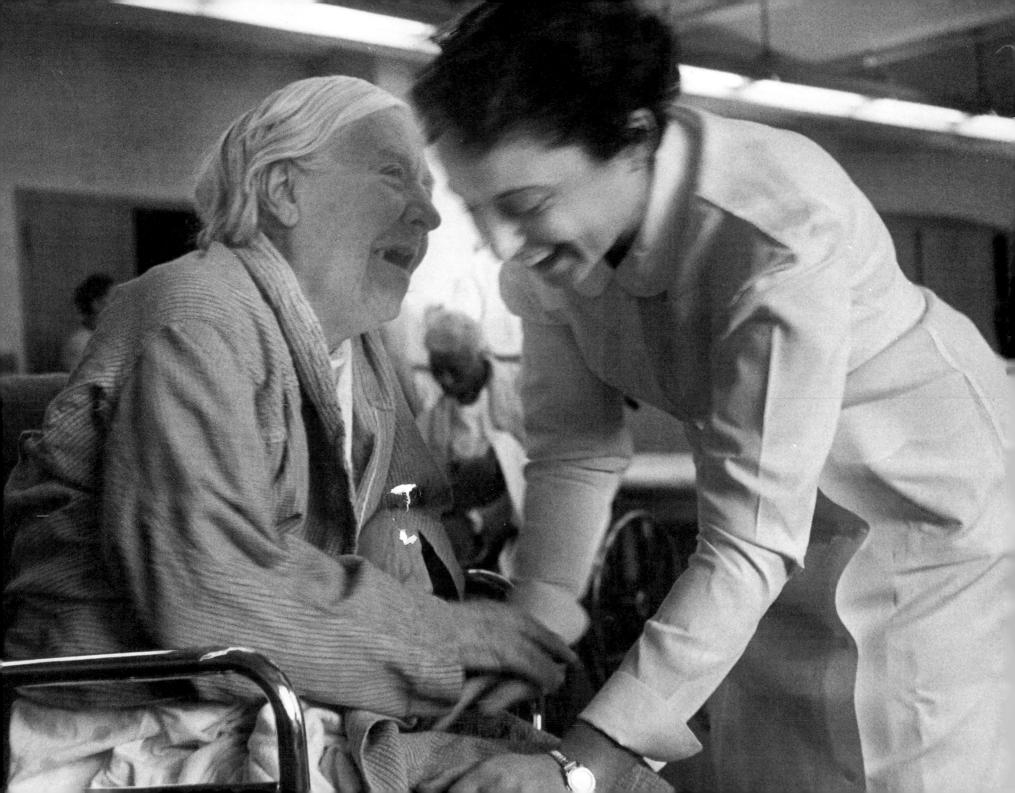

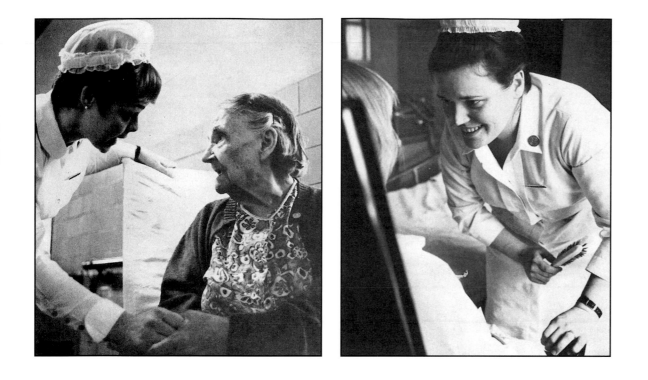

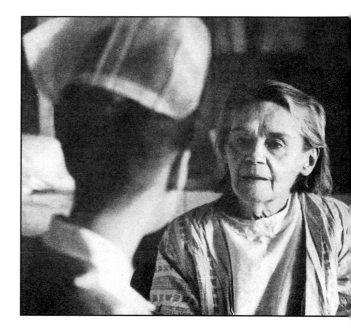

"*It's hard work. As hard as that on the surgical floor. There's never enough of me to go around. I say this humbly; there's never enough of any nurse to go around. Is the geriatric patient ever truly comfortable, or truly unafraid? The needs are always there; they go on and on after I'm sure that I cannot. But geriatric nursing is never dull—never! After each shift at the nursing home, I find myself terribly tired and serenely satisfied.*"

FRANCIS STORLIE

DECEMBER 1965

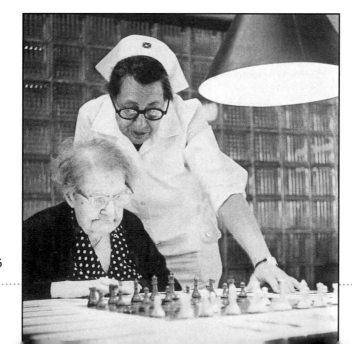

Mrs. Reynolds Needs a Nurse

Mrs. Reynolds was a real patient at Harborview Hospital in Seattle. And the story told about her and the nurses who cared for her in the film *Mrs. Reynolds Needs a Nurse* is told just the way it happened. Produced with an educational fund from Smith, Kline, and French, this film was a nursing school "classic" in the 1960s and 1970s. Dolores Little, the supervisor in the film and in the real-life situation, is shown, standing, in the lower left photo.

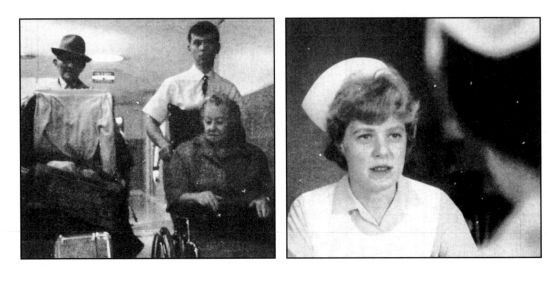

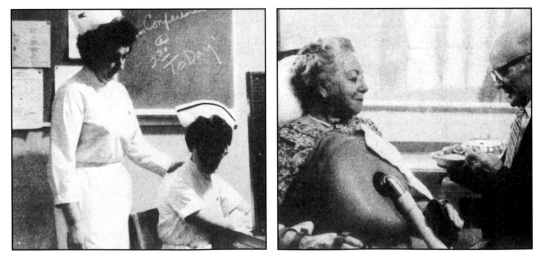

Mrs. Reynolds arrives on the busy, overcrowded ward. She is very ill, frightened, demanding—dependent on her husband and "things" for security. A student cannot accept that the kind of nursing she is learning about cannot be given on a busy ward. Her protests—and her understanding—convince her supervisor. The supervisor consults a psychiatric nursing instructor on how to bring about the necessary changes on Mrs. Reynolds' ward—in staff attitudes, staff behavior. The Head Nurse's resistance was to be expected—she was short-handed. Mr. Reynolds got under foot and broke the rules. But in the end she, too, tried. Change came. Mrs. Reynolds changed; so did her husband when he was taught how to help. And the new way yielded a happier patient and staff.

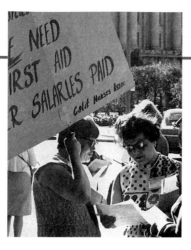

Commentary

Anne Zimmerman

Economic Justice

Nurses have traditionally struggled with low pay and long working hours. In its early years, the ANA had focused its attention on activities deemed essential to nursing's becoming a profession, but it did acknowledge the serious economic hardship most nurses faced. Although there was talk about the financial issue in some state nurses associations, mostly in New York and California, it was not until 1914 that ANA President Genevieve Cooke directly asked the delegates to think seriously about challenging the economic insecurity faced by those in the profession.

During the Great Depression, nurses suffered along with others. The ANA issued a statement for inclusion in President Franklin Roosevelt's National Recovery Act of 1933, which advocated an eight-hour work day and 48-hour work week for nurses. During this time, nurses' registries were studied and standards were established for private duty nurses working in homes and in the community.

During World War II, nurses siphoned off by the military created a shortage of health care professionals in civilian institutions. The War Labor Board had frozen salaries, leaving nurses grossly underpaid. Many left the profession for more lucrative wartime jobs, worsening an already serious situation.

It was the determination of Shirley Titus, the Executive Director of the California State Nurses Association (later CNA), that led to the establishment of the first statewide salary for staff nurses, enabling a successful approach to the War Labor Board, which allowed an increase in nurses' salaries. Based upon this success, CNA moved quickly to represent nurses with employers, and it was this, together with similar activities in several other states, that stimulated the 1946 ANA House of Delegates to adopt an economic security program that included collective bargaining. This was a landmark decision for nursing.

During this same time, at a preconvention meeting of the delegates, a platform spelling out what the ANA stood for was accepted. This platform included work toward full adoption of an eight-hour day (which had been established in 1934) and a 40-hour work week with no decrease in salary; participation in social security; and support for the idea of nurses' professional associations acting as their exclusive spokesperson.

From 1936 to 1947, nurses and other workers were covered by the National Labor Relations Act (NLRA), which protected employees' rights to organize and bargain collectively. The passage of the Taft-Hartley Act in 1947, however, posed a serious deterrent to organizing. Although private and non-profit hospitals were not precluded from recognizing and bargaining with an employee association, they were not required to; thus the rights of nurses and other hospital workers were not protected. Nevertheless, nurses pushed on and pursued voluntary recognition and collective bargaining agreements. They were aided by considerable media support; leadership from highly respected nurses who committed their energies to the program; mass resignations in lieu of strikes; and, in 1966, the rescinding of the 1950 ANA no-strike clause, which nurses had naively believed would persuade employers to be responsive to their rights.

In 1962, President John F. Kennedy issued an executive order protecting the collective bargaining rights of nurses and others employed in federal hospitals. This, together with state labor laws and the establishment of a national salary goal in 1966, all helped to advance nursing's goals for representation and a better way of life. In 1974, after a 27-year battle to gain protection for nurses under the NLRA, Congress amended the Taft-Hartley Act, removing the exemption that nonprofits enjoyed. Unfortunately, this long-sought success was a mixed blessing, bringing increased and more sophisticated opposition by employers. They challenged, among other things, the composition of the organization as a legitimate labor organization and whether an all RN unit was appropriate under law. Frequently, the expensive services of antiunion firms were retained by employers.

Despite all this, there were court decisions that favored nurses, and state nurses associations such as those in California, New York, Ohio, Minnesota, Michigan, Pennsylvania, and Illinois moved ahead vigorously to represent

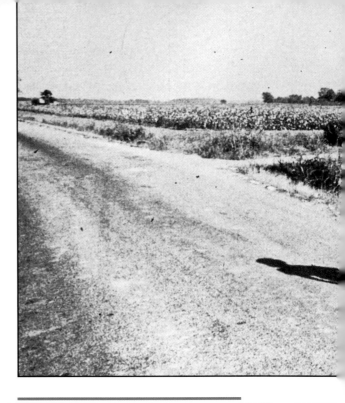

Nurses fight dust and distances in the rural South.

"...*h*ow do you measure the debilitating, demoralizing effects of poverty, the erosion of strength, the progressive deterioration of bones, muscles, and tissues from years of malnutrition, hard work, and neglect? How do you measure defeated hopes, lost resources, weariness of soul?"

MARION MOSES, UNITED FARM WORKERS
NOVEMBER 1969

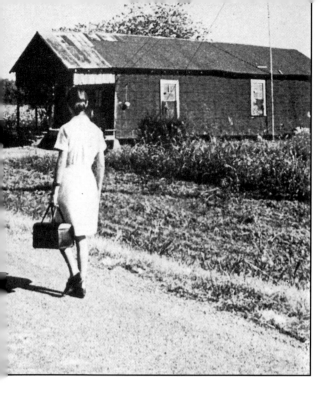

nurses. In states where there was no collective bargaining through the state nurses association, the ANA Work Place Advocacy program has been effective in assisting nurses.

It was not only the legal obstacles and employer resistance that stood in the way of successful organizing for nurses. Through the years, the concept of organizing has been anathema to some nurses who feel it is "unprofessional." Fear of strikes by nurses is often raised, although they have been few, and when they have occurred, nursing care has always been provided for patients in need. Nurses who actively exercise their right to representation and a voice in patient care and employment security have more access to the way decisions are made, but all nurses and nursing benefit from their efforts.

Nurse-midwife Sister Mary Stella started a prenatal clinic in a storefront.

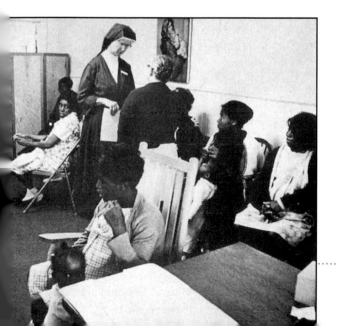

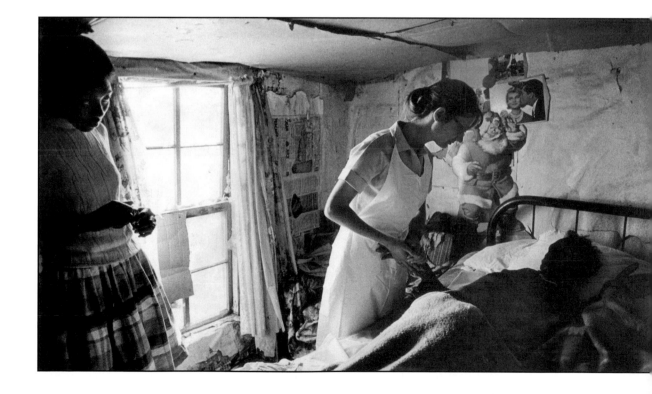

"The issue at stake is not just better salaries, pensions, vacations, et cetera. The real issue is who shall control nursing, nursing practice, nursing quality. . . . Nurses have permitted an erosion of both their rights and their responsibilities to result from their employment situation in the modern hospital. This is a failure in public service on the part of nurses at every level: the leaders who stand aloof; the academic nurses who are willing to wait for the next generation; the directors of diploma schools and of hospital nursing service departments who are unwilling to jeopardize their position with management; the rank and file who don't want to be bothered, who can't find any reserves of courage, who won't spend the money, who will not think. Sometimes I believe we are a sorry lot—but most of the time I think we just haven't learned how to loose the bonds of tradition."

DOROTHY KELLY
on Collective Bargaining
JANUARY 1965

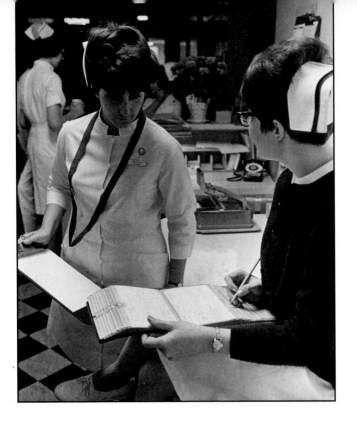

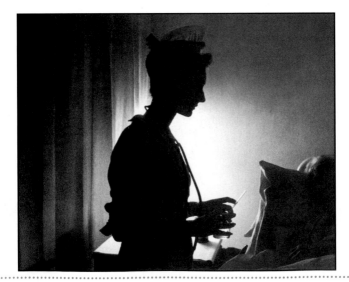

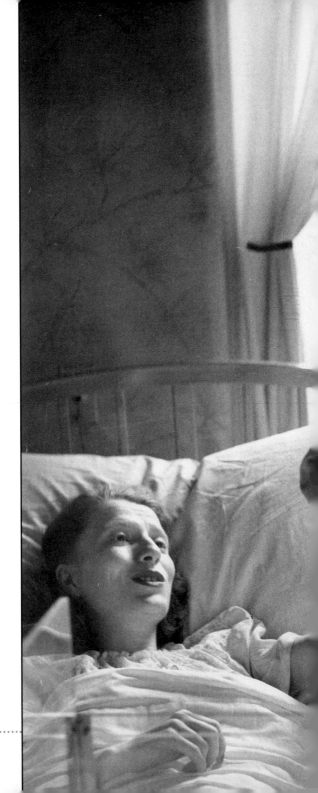

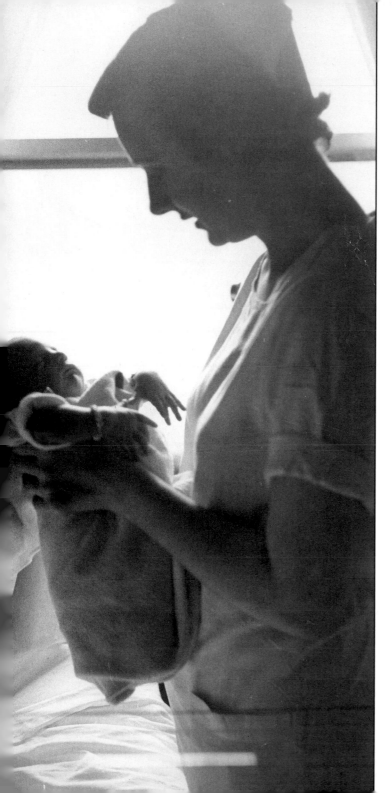

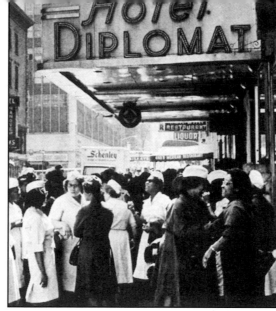

In May of 1966, almost half of the nurses of New York City's municipal hospitals were prepared to resign over poor working conditions and low salaries. Lengthy negotiations between the city and the New York State Nurses Association, the bargaining agent for the nurses, resulted in an agreement in time to prevent the resignations.

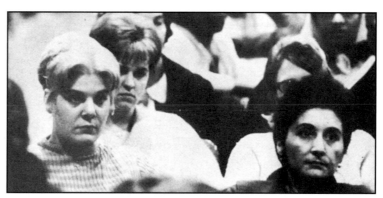

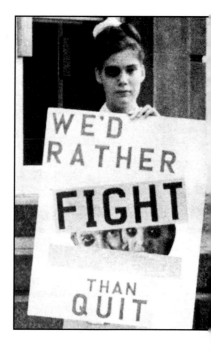

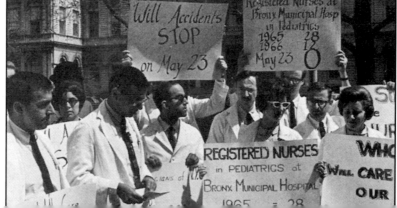

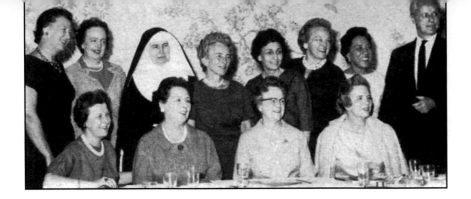

First steps in a comprehensive study of nursing education was planned by the ANA-NLN Committee on Conference. Standing (left to right): Rena Boyle, NLN staff; Margaret F. Carroll, ANA staff; Sister Maureen, ANA Board; Lucile P. Leone, NLN Board; Minnie H. Walton, NLN staff; Jo Eleanor Elliott, ANA Board; Willetta Simonton, ANA staff; Robert K. Merton, ANA consulting sociologist. Seated: Judith G. Whitaker, ANA executive director; Ines Haynes, NLN general director; Lois M. Austin, NLN president; Margaret B. Dolan, ANA president.

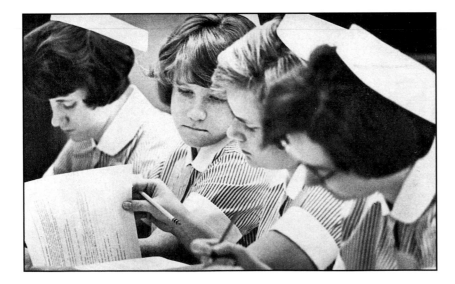

The question of how nursing students were to be educated was hotly debated, and in 1965, the ANA called for baccalaureate education as the basic foundation for professional nursing.

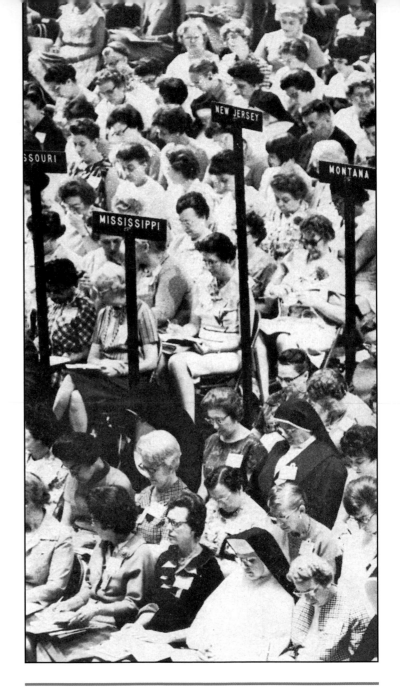

Delegates at the 1966 ANA convention are serious, pondering the impact on nursing of their decisions.

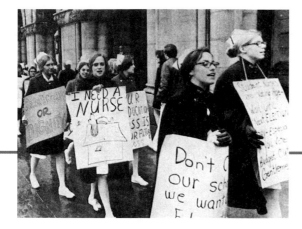

Changing Times, Changing Roles

1970–1979

Political issues were prominent in the 1970s, and nurses, mirroring the country's population, were divided. The Vietnam War, the Equal Rights Amendment, national health insurance, abortion, the women's movement—all issues that found as many nurses on the right as on the left, with many silent in the middle. During this decade, nurses spoke up for peace, human rights, civil rights, and for rights to fair salaries and working conditions. They sought autonomy in their profession and a voice in governance.

During the 1970s, nursing was plagued with internal divisions over professional issues. The advance of the nurse practitioner movement stirred anger in those who believed primary care by nurses was "junior doctoring." Repeal in 1974 of the Taft-Hartley Amendment that had exempted nonprofit hospitals from having to bargain with employees spurred the American Nurses Association and its state associations to intensify their efforts, offending many nurses in management. "Entry into practice" arguments also continued to rage.

But the 1970s were also a time of introspection. Death and dying were prominent themes, and the writings of Elizabeth Kubler-Ross, Cicely Saunders, and Sister Madeleine Clémence Vaillot forced people—especially nurses—to think about their personal responses. By the end of the decade, out of the dissension and contemplation, there emerged a growing sense of self-worth among nurses and a new understanding of their caring function by the public.

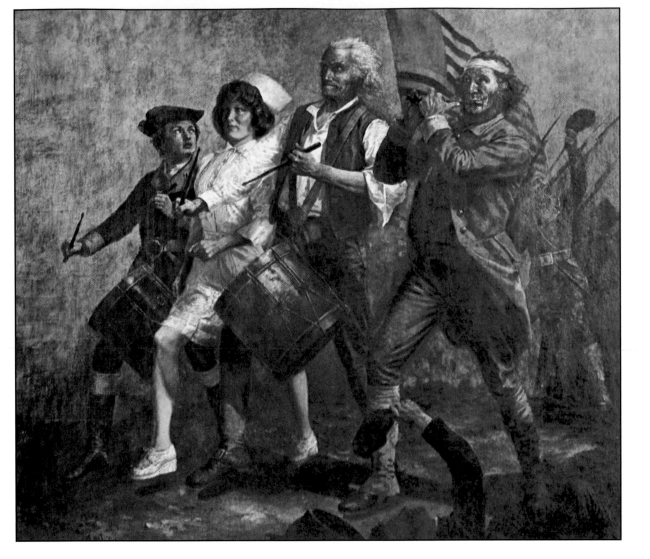

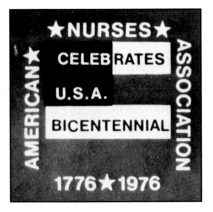

COMMENT

All over this country, there are nurses
with keen brains and good skills going to waste because
they're putting all their cognitive energy into ruminating
on what's wrong with the state of our art. It's time to stop
worrying about Sairey Gamp and start identifying with
Lavinia Dock. We have a sore need today for genuine
heroes and heroines. The Bicentennial reminds us that we
have them.   APRIL, 1975

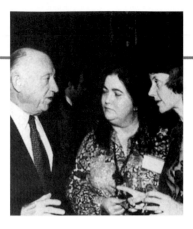

Commentary

Constance Holleran

The American Nurses Association and the Art of Politics

The American Nurses Association (ANA) has played an active role in the enactment of health laws and related social legislation for many years. For the first half of the century, volunteers monitored hearings in Washington and scanned the Congressional Record alerting the ANA to significant bills, speeches, and hearings of interest to nursing. By the 1950s, activity in Washington warranted the opening of a small, one-person office, which was staffed by Julia Thompson, RN.

During the 1960s, health legislation suddenly became controversial when the question of Medicare arose. The ANA had a very active part in working for Medicare enactment, enough so that in 1965, ANA President Jo Eleanor Elliott and Julia Thompson were taken on the presidential plane to the Truman Library in Independence, Missouri, for the signing of that significant piece of legislation.

Life seemed much less complicated in Washington in the 1960s. For example, the Secretary of Health, Education, and Welfare would routinely call the ANA Washington office to see whom it wanted to have named to commissions and committees being appointed.

This changed drastically in the 1970s and 1980s. In 1970, the ANA Washington office was staffed with two nurses and one secretary. ANA headquarters were in New York City, and the Washington climate for health groups was getting cooler. As a result, a group of nurse leaders approached ANA leadership and argued for a stronger presence in Washington in order to ensure adequate legislative support for the upcoming extension of the Nurse Training Act and for appropriations for various other health programs.

It was agreed that personnel would be added to the Washington ANA office, and in January 1971, I assumed the directorship, as Julia Thompson was retiring. Other nursing organizations continued to work cooperatively with the ANA on legislation. Gradually the office space was expanded.

Direct contact with every nursing school was initiated, and that, plus frequent, "quick action" memos to all state nurses associations, resulted in a high profile for nursing on Capitol Hill. Staff were hired to work with Executive Branch agencies as they drafted proposals and worked on regulations for various programs. Another part of the job was to be sure the ANA received early warning signals on upcoming issues and plans.

The position was also educational to staff members of Congress. Duties included monitoring, urging changes in drafts, preparing, and, at times, presenting testimony, and attending all work sessions where congressional committees made final decisions. On occasion, with the chairperson's permission, it was essential to speak up openly on a point.

As ANA leadership was not ready to start a political action committee (PAC) to support political candidates in the mid-1970s, a group of nurses in the New York area formed a small organization to fill that gap. The director of the Washington office of the ANA informally advised them and put them in touch with other health professional PAC groups. In time, that group and the ANA worked in a united fashion, and the Nurses Coalition for Action in Politics (N-CAP) was formed as the political action arm of the ANA. (It is now called ANA PAC.)

Staff with experience in grass roots organizing and working with Congress were brought on. Great care was taken to coordinate the legislative and political arms of the ANA office and to abide by federal campaign laws. Fund-raising was surprisingly slow, but campaign volunteers were plentiful as things got rolling.

The Washington office organized legislative workshops and Congressional receptions. ANA members who came to Washington for these events were fully briefed and sessions were arranged with their own elected congressional delegations, as a group or individually, to discuss legislative con-

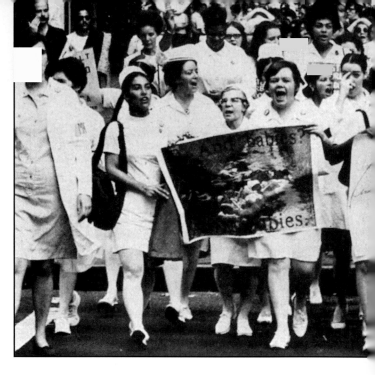

Nurses March for Peace, Start National Group

*N*EW YORK, NY—*Down Fifth Avenue on May 23, nurses were on the march—not for pay and not for a greater voice in patient care, but in protest against U.S. involvement in Southeast Asia. About 500 nurses, many of them in uniform, walked down the avenue at a fast pace, smiling, singing, "All we are saying is give peace a chance," and carrying signs reading, "Thou shalt not kill to honor America." Their march and subsequent rally were sponsored by Nurses for Peace, an anti-war group that had its inception at New York University.*

JULY, 1970

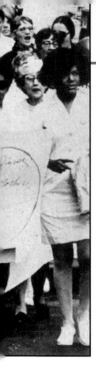

"Life, not death"—"We shall overcome"—"Give peace a chance," nurse marchers chorused.

"All nurses stand for peace, in the world and in the hearts of men. The stand taken by the professional organization at the ANA Convention in Miami makes it clear that nurses support interests directed toward peace. Nurses everywhere have a long and proud tradition that supports preservation of life and promotion of healthy living. Nurses will continue to accept and act upon this social responsibility."

HILDEGARD E. PEPLAU, President,
American Nurses' Association,
JULY 1970

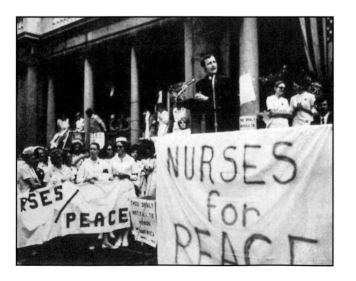

cerns. Meetings in the district offices were also helpful. Nursing was united on legislation.

ANA staff also worked extensively in a leadership role with other groups, such as the Coalition for Health Funding and the Mental Health Centers working group. Together they spearheaded a number of successful veto overrides for important health bills and health appropriations.

The cooperation and coordination between the ANA, the National League for Nursing (NLN), and the American Association of Colleges of Nursing (AACN) were essential for success in those years. The ANA conducted its first public opinion poll to determine where its members stood on various social and other public policy issues. While many members were conservative on issues such as defense, there was wide support for federal assistance for many aspects of health policy. This information guided the N-CAP and ANA Board in decision making. Policies for the N-CAP candidate endorsement process were also agreed upon. Key legislative issues were identified and health-related voting records of all members of Congress were tabulated, published, and used in determining which candidates were to be supported. The state nurses associations had to agree to any endorsement of candidates from their states.

Soon, states began to organize PACs, and fund raising events were held at each ANA convention. The first, a luncheon which featured Alan Alda of M*A*S*H fame (a great supporter of women's rights), was a sell-out.

Today, nursing has a few of its own in the House of Representatives. Although there are none yet in the Senate, there are many supporters of this endeavor in Washington and across the nation. It will not be long.

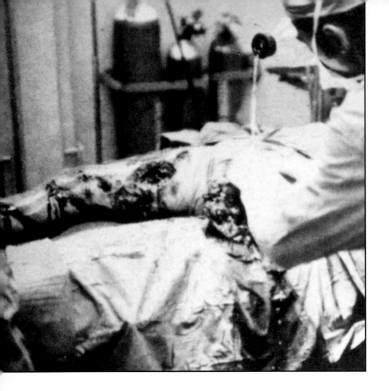

In Southeast Asia, the war raged on.

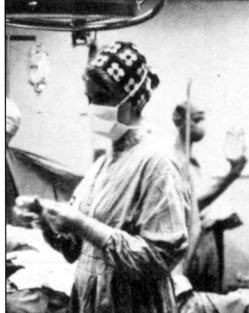

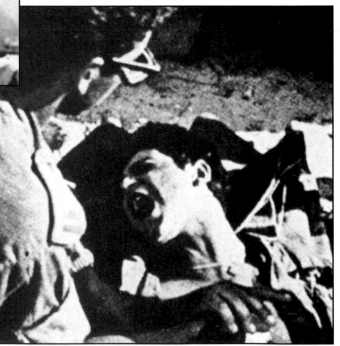

It is terribly hard, after being so involved with war and its tragedy, to forget or even to push it aside to a corner of one's mind. Memories of the boys and men we patched back together and who subsequently lived are overshadowed by all those we couldn't "fix," all those who later died, and all those who later wished they had died.

Someday this will end and I'll go home and wear cute white uniforms and work an eight-hour day and sleep without nightmares, and I'll be happy and satisfied with a hospital pediatric ward job and I'll forget I ever lived in this horror and who are you trying to kid anyway, Jones?

NANCY JONES, JULY 1971

Letters

Several months ago a young man in my town was wounded in action in Vietnam and died a short time later. Relatively soon after this his young wife received a letter from one of the nurses who cared for him during his hospital stay, and I in turn wrote to the nurse to ask permission to share her letter with others. The letter follows:

Perhaps I am stepping a bit out of line to write to you now at the time of your sorrow and soul-shattering grief. However, I felt I wanted you to know how very, very brave your young husband was, even as ill as he was.

I am an Army nurse and have only been in Vietnam a little over a month. I still find it most difficult to see our young men suffer as they do. Your husband made a very definite spot in each of our hearts. He was sweet, kind and patient with us—even if he had a wait of a few minutes while we cared for the other 49 patients on our ward. When he passed away, we all felt a very minute part of the grief you must feel. His passing was quiet and quite painless, if that is any comfort to you.

It was my job to clean his table and it was there I found your address. I'm sorry I don't even know your first name but I took what was in the corner of the envelope. I kept thinking of you and what you would go through in the next few days and nights. I came home and wept bitterly and prayed that it might not be too hard for you. I don't know why I feel this way because we were taught long ago not to become attached to our patients, their families or their problems. But I guess my Christian upbringing has taught me, there is such a thing as love and concern for our fellow man.

Please don't feel it is necessary you to write, as I'm sure that will be the last thing on your mind. Just accept this as my poor way of expressing my deepest sympathy to you, and may God be especially close to you through all this, as he obviously was with your husband.

I can't tell you how much this letter moved me and how much it meant to his family. It made me proud of my profession and of those nurses who gave of themselves voluntarily in military service to provide the best care for the young men.

Jean T. Lassiter, RN
June 1970

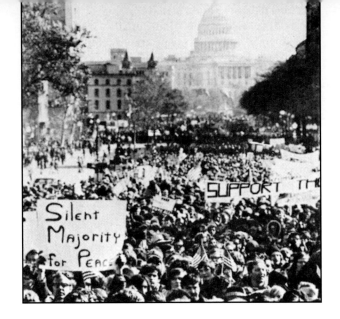

Moratorium Day in Washington, DC, when Americans from all over the country came together for a peace march. The war would not end, however, until 1973 when President Richard Nixon ordered a halt to all offensive military operations against North Vietnam.

Nurses on the march . . .

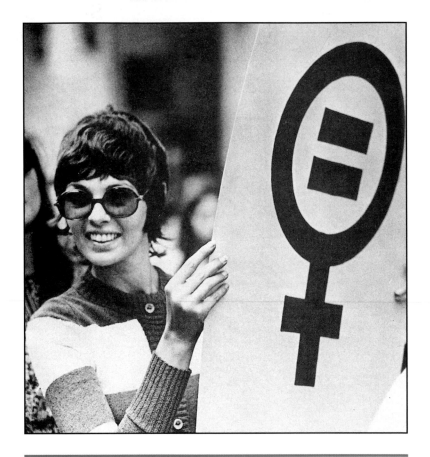

They marched for women's rights . . .

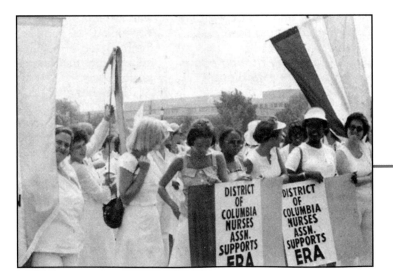

Nurses were well represented in the crowd of 100,000 that gathered in Washington to support extension of the ratification deadline for the Equal Rights Amendment. Most of the participants in the march wore white, just as the suffragettes did 65 years ago.

They marched for patients' rights . . .

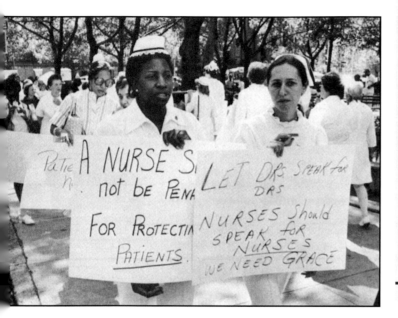

Denver Nurses Charge Sex Discrimination in Pay Scales

*D*ENVER, CO—*Nine nurses employed by the Denver Hospital and Visiting Nurse Service recently filed a class-action in U.S. Federal District Court of Colorado for all nurses employed by the city and county of Denver. The suit challenged widespread sex discrimination against nurses and the undervaluation of nurses' services. Right, three of the nine registered nurses who filed the suit in 1977.*

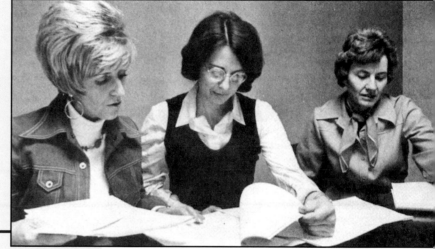

They marched for nurses' rights.

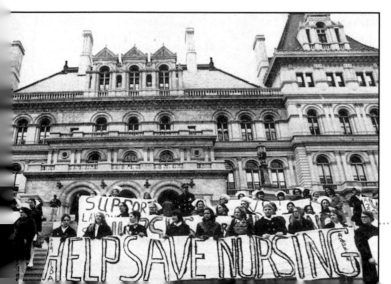

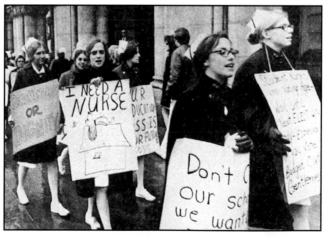

White caps on the capitol steps in Albany—several thousand nurses took part in the demonstration.

*W*e *have done little to assert our right to an independent practice and to stake our claim to that part of health care which is ours. True, we have screamed aloud or writhed secretly, according to our individual natures, about being referred to as "handmaidens." But we have failed to work constructively to change the system which perpetuates this stereotype. So, I would say to nurses facetiously, and yet sincerely: Handmaidens of the world, arise!*

AVA DILWORTH, RN
FEBRUARY, 1971

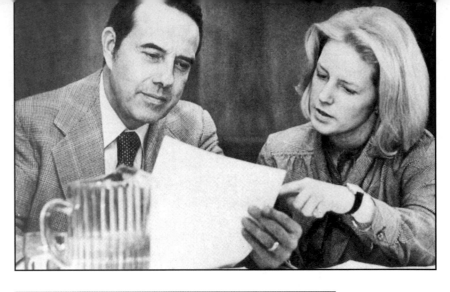

Nurse Training Provisions Pass Over Presidential Veto

*W*ASHINGTON, DC—*The months of struggle on the part of Congress and health groups have borne fruit, and federal health programs—including those for nursing—will be continued in spite of a presidential veto.*

ANA's Constance Holleran discusses strategy with Senator Edward Kennedy following the veto override.

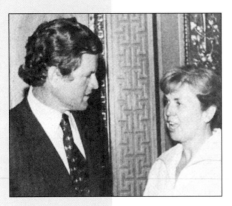

SEPTEMBER, 1975

Sheila Burke makes a point about a piece of health legislation to Senator Robert Dole, for whom she is a staff aide.

Rhetaugh Dumas Is Deputy at Institute of Mental Health

*W*ASHINGTON, DC—*Department of Health, Education and Welfare has named a psychiatric nurse to be deputy director of the National Institute of Mental Health.*

Rhetaugh Dumas, RN, MSN, PhD., now has the highest rank of any psychiatric nurse in government.

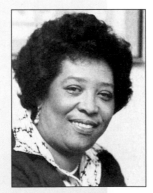

DECEMBER, 1979

Senator/nurse Rosalie Abrams was also chairperson of the Maryland Democratic Central Committee. A member of the Maryland House of Delegates in 1967, she won her state senate seat in 1970.

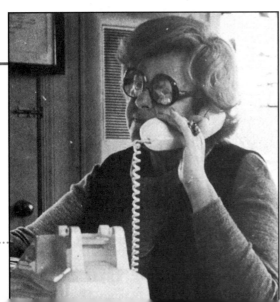

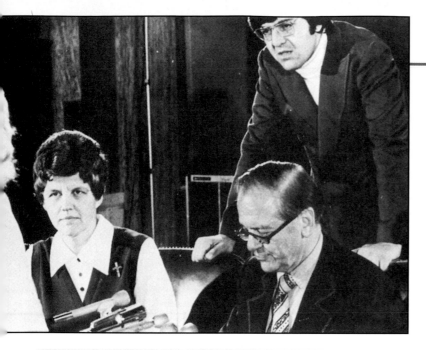

Hearing a questioner at the public briefing on long-term care is Sister Marilyn Schwab (ANA spokesperson). With her are Senator Moss (seated) and Val J. Halamandaris, majority staff member for the Moss subcommittee.

First Lady and Chairperson of the President's Commission on Mental Health Rosalynn Carter is flanked by ANA President Barbara Nichols (left) and Martha Mitchell, Chairperson of ANA's Commission on Psychiatric and Mental Health Nursing Practice and member of the President's Commission at D.C. General Hospital.

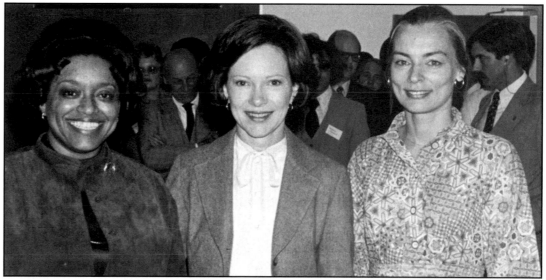

Nurse Heads National Rape Advisory Committee

*C*HESTNUT HILL, MA—*Ann Burgess, RN, who co-founded one of the nation's first rape victim counseling programs at Boston City Hospital in 1972, now heads a new 12-member Rape Prevention and Control Advisory Committee. The Committee, appointed by former HEW Secretary David Mathews, will advise the National Center for the Prevention and Control of Rape.*

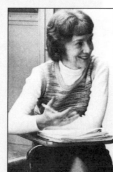

MARCH, 1977

Joy Ufema, RN, studied thanatology for two years and became a specialist in the care of dying patients and their families. Her career was highlighted on television, first on *Sixty Minutes* and then in an hour-long docudrama.

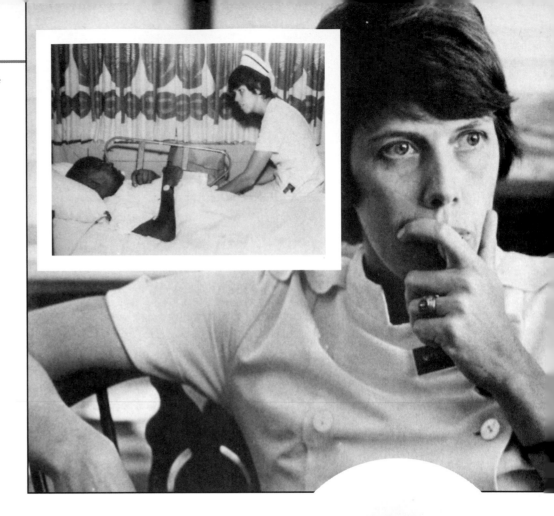

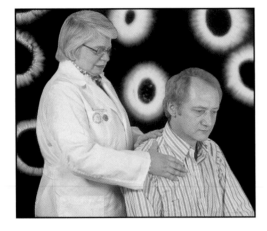

Dr. Dolores Krieger pioneered and researched therapeutic touch as a healing method within the scope of nursing practice.

*D*are to care for the dying . . .
"I am a staff nurse who works in the specialty area of death and dying. Strange as it may seem. I love it."

JOY UFEMA, RN
JANUARY, 1976

Two of the first group of nurses who achieved certification in clinical practice.

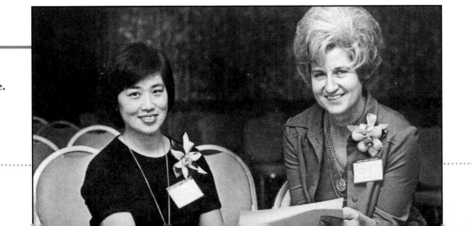

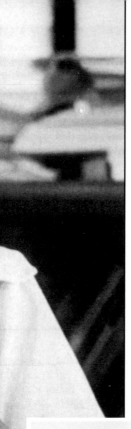

When M. Lucille Kinlein, RN, MS, hung out her shingle as an independent nurse practitioner in 1971, she became a role model for the many who since have followed.

When Loeb Center for Nursing and Rehabilitation, Montefiore Hospital, New York City, opened its doors to patients, its primary purpose was to demonstrate that high quality nursing care given solely by registered nurses, in a nondirective setting, offered a supportive service to people in the postacute phase of their illness that enabled them to recover sooner, and to leave the center able to cope with themselves and what they must face in the future.

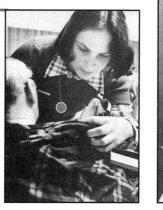

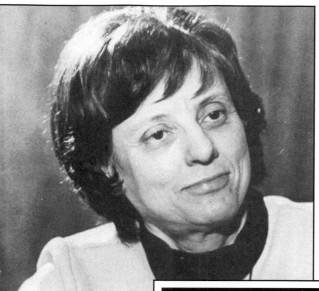

M. LUCILLE KINLEIN, RN
INDEPENDENT
GENERALIST NURSE

Audra Pambrun was named the ANA's "most involved nurse" for 1970, culminating a nationwide search conducted as part of the "BE-INVOLVED" program sponsored by Schering Laboratories. She is shown here with fellow Montanan, Senator Mike Mansfield. Miss Pambrun, the second Blackfoot Indian ever to become an RN, established the first suicide crisis intervention center for Blackfeet Indians. Her district is over 1 million acres, her caseload almost 7,000 Blackfeet. She gave half of her $2,000 award to the center.
JULY, 1970

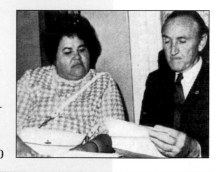

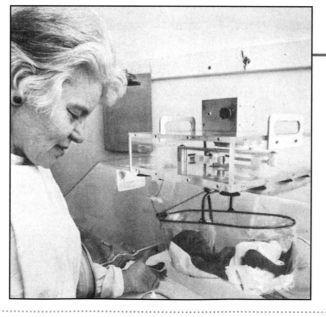

Incubator hammock, which gives the premature infant a rocking motion similar to motion in the womb, is checked by Mary V. Neal, associate professor and chairman of pediatric nursing at the University of Maryland School of Nursing, who devised it as part of her doctoral studies at New York University.

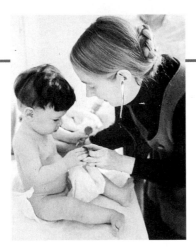

Commentary

Claire Fagin

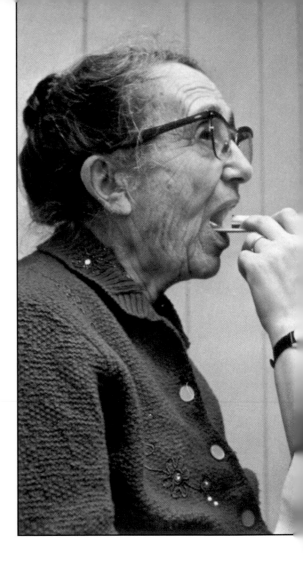

Progress and Maturity in Education and Practice

Nursing, a profession of promise and paradox, is at once thrilling and frustrating. It is a profession of in-touchness with people, yet it is often misunderstood or un-understood by them. It has made extraordinary progress during this century of its formalization, yet it has been unable to come to grips with its educational dilemma—the one ingredient that would solidify its progress.

Today we see nurses at policy tables throughout the world in health ministries, as presidents and provosts of colleges and universities, on corporate boards, and on important governmental commissions. From my perspective there have been defining moments during this century that denote progress and maturity, with the underlying theme being the historical linkage between education and practice. These successful and lasting milestones include the development of public health nursing, and Lillian Wald's establishment of the Henry Street Settlement on the Lower East Side of New York; the development of critical care nursing, which changed the face of hospital nursing; the nurse practitioner movement—from primary to tertiary care—which included the formalization of higher education for nurse-midwives; the integration of nursing education and nursing practice in many settings; the federal approval of nursing's accreditation of clinical care through the Community Health Accreditation Program; and the development of educational programs and practice and research opportunities for advanced practice nurses. Reimbursement from public and private payers

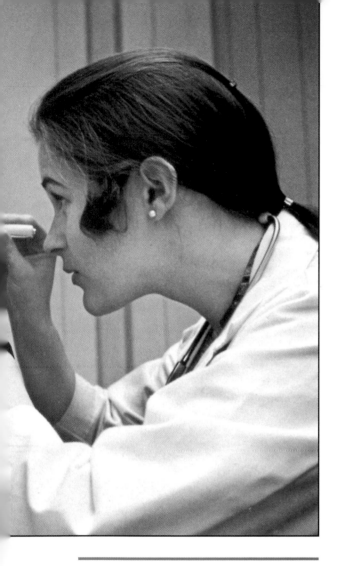

Nurse practitioners work in all kinds of settings, with all kinds of patients.

seemed an impossible dream at many points during the past few decades, but this too was accomplished.

I see the development of the clinical specialist, now referred to as the advanced practice nurse, as one of the most dramatic contemporary occurrences in nursing. The advanced practice nurse has become institutionalized and is recognized as useful, effective, and highly valuable. This grew from the need for highly skilled nurses to work knowledgeably with specialized populations, given the burgeoning knowledge in the medical field. Once this need was recognized, advanced practice nursing received significant support from the federal government, foundations, and institutional leadership.

Progress and maturity in nursing over the past 25 years can also be seen in individual instances. For example, nurses came together to support Nursing's Agenda for Health Care Reform, crafted by the ANA and endorsed by more than 60 other nursing organizations. Led by Pamela Maraldo and Maria Mitchell at the National League for Nursing, and Carolyne Davis, the Community Health Accreditation Program (CHAP), nursing's accrediting body for home care companies, was granted deemed status by the Health Care Financing Administration in 1992. Thus, CHAP-accredited agencies automatically qualified for federal reimbursement under Medicare and Medicaid.

The historic significance of this achievement for nursing and health care cannot be underestimated. It was the first time a nursing organization had been given the right to determine the practice standards for a whole sector of the health care system, an event we can only hope to replicate in other areas with more widespread use of the Magnet Hospital designation. CHAP also committed to a policy of full public disclosure of health care information and included consumers in its governance structure and boards of review. CHAP set a gold standard.

Where nursing has not set a gold standard is in its apparent inability to resolve the question of entry into the profession. The current and future demand for advanced practice nurses is predicated on a supply of baccalaureate-prepared nurses eligible for entry to masters level programs. Yet, we are seeing a reduction in their numbers. The diverse educational entry points that nursing offers are commendable; however, diversity on entry should not be confused with diversity on completion of requirements for registration for the RN license. This was never the intention of the leaders who developed associate degree programs. They conceived of the program as replacing the dominant hospital diploma course and providing a differentiating credential from the baccalaureate.

As a whole, the nursing profession has responded to change with sensitivity and flexibility, all the while keeping nursing's historical mission of caring and concern for the public's health in direct focus. Evidence of nursing's proactive stance with regard to progress includes rapid changes in educational programs at the baccalaureate and higher degree levels to prepare for practice in primary care, a greater focus on clinical skills at all levels, investment in training for faculty research and practice, and studies on the cost effectiveness of many nursing interventions.

Nursing's record in responding to mandates for change is exemplary. Leadership of nursing educators in the overarching scene of health care, encouraging, conducting, and publicizing research on effects of changing practices on patient care, and affecting local and national health care policies are necessary actions for now and into the new century.

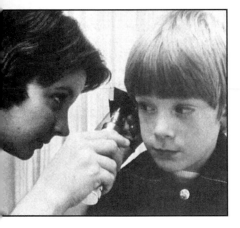

Nurse practitioner and her patient in a rural health clinic.

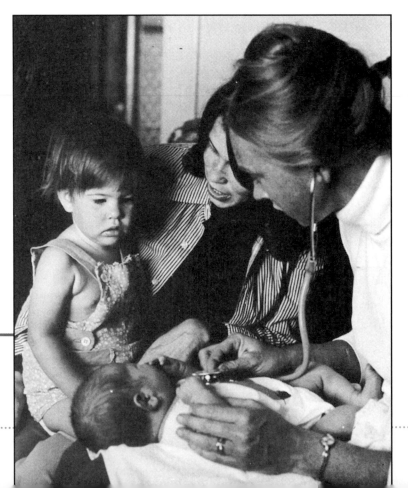

Neonatal nurse practitioner visits mothers and babies who were discharged within 24 hours.

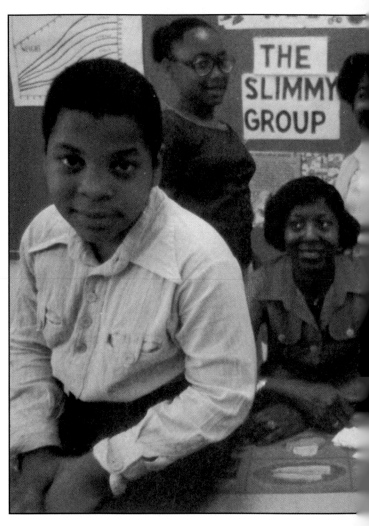

School nurse practitioner with a children's weight control group.

144

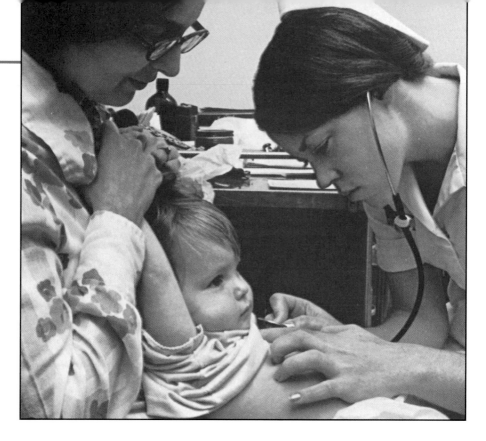

Pediatric nurse practitioner examines a baby at an army base clinic.

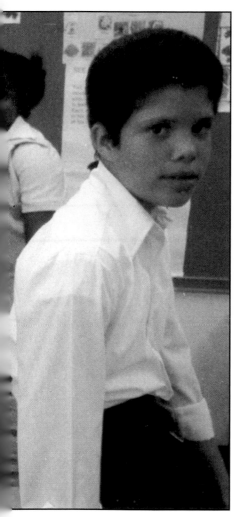

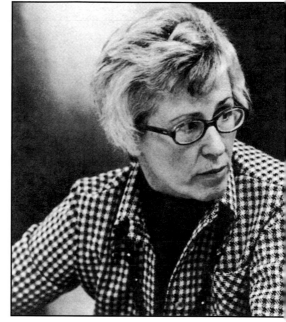

Loretta C. Ford, cofounder of the original pediatric nurse practitioner program in Colorado.

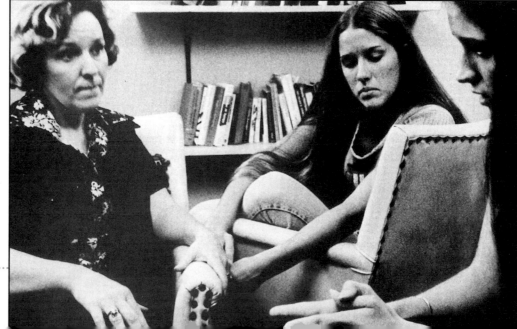

Psychiatric/mental health nurse specialist counsels teenagers.

145

Nurses took patients' health care concerns to heart and were in the vanguard of changing the way health care is provided, and to whom.

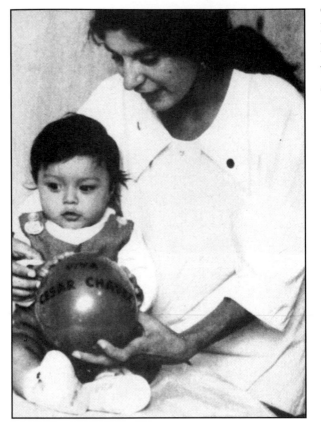

"What people need most when they are dying is relief from distressing symptoms of disease, the security of a caring environment, sustained expert care, and assurance that they and their families will not be abandoned."

JOAN CRAVEN AND
FLORENCE S. WALD
OCTOBER 1975

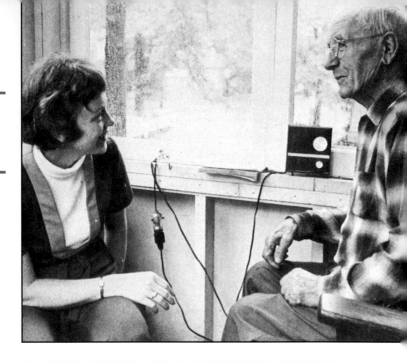

Hospice care begins with listening.

During the grape strike in California, Marion Moses volunteered to help provide health care for strikers and their families. She went for a month and remained for five years, working with Cesar Chavez and the United Farm Workers.

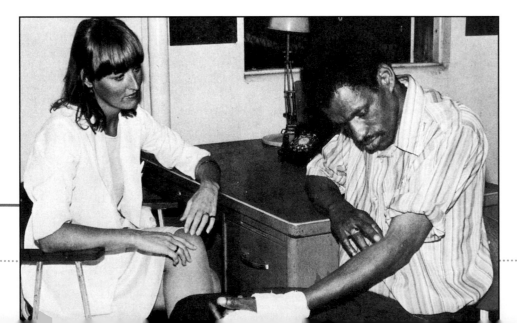

Gail Pisarcik sees a patient in the ER. For some patients, this is their only contact with a mental health professional.

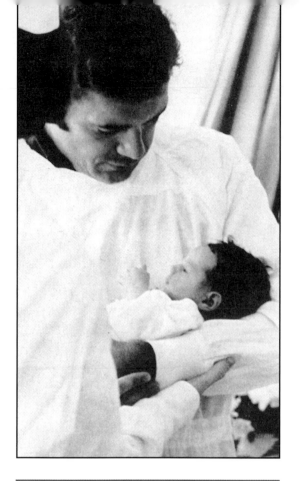

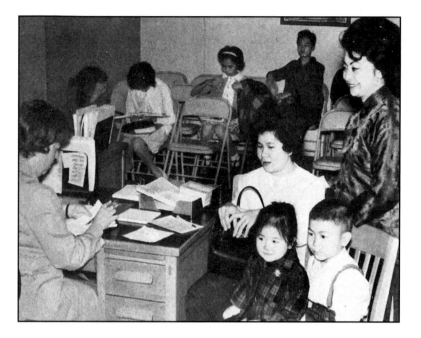

Interviewing a family at a TB clinic in San Francisco's Chinatown.

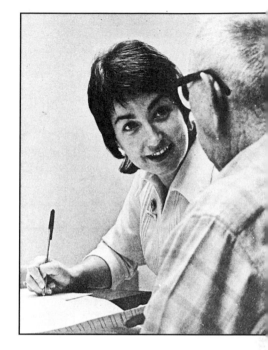

A Minnesota nurse practitioner in an urban high-rise housing unit for the elderly.

Mercy Hospital in Miami was among the small but growing number of hospitals in this country where a father was not restricted to regular visiting hours—he was not a visitor, but an integral part of the family unit.

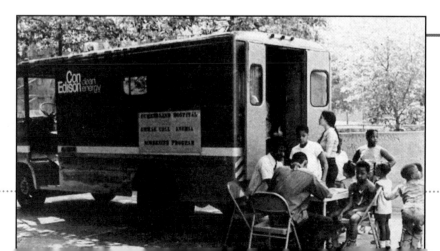

Using vans on loan from the electric company, nurses brought care to the people—wherever they were. Cumberland Hospital staff go into a Brooklyn, New York community to test for sickle cell anemia.

147

Despite the marches, the turmoil, the struggles for professional and personal identity, the one constant was caring.

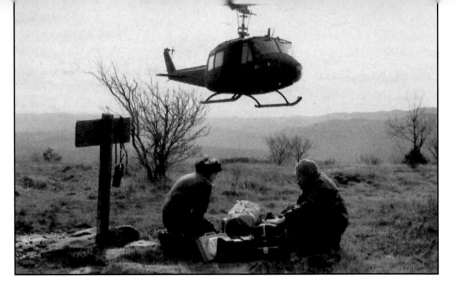

After being brought by helicopter to the top of a 6,000-foot mountain in the Great Smokies, volunteer nurses prepared to hike to the scene of an airplane crash.

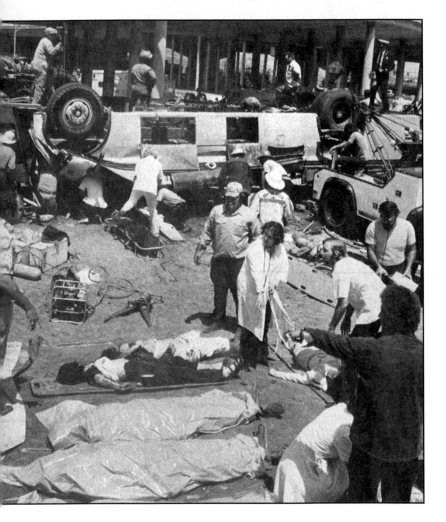

Nurses examine a boating accident victim on his arrival at the dock built by Point Pleasant (NJ) Hospital for just such purposes.

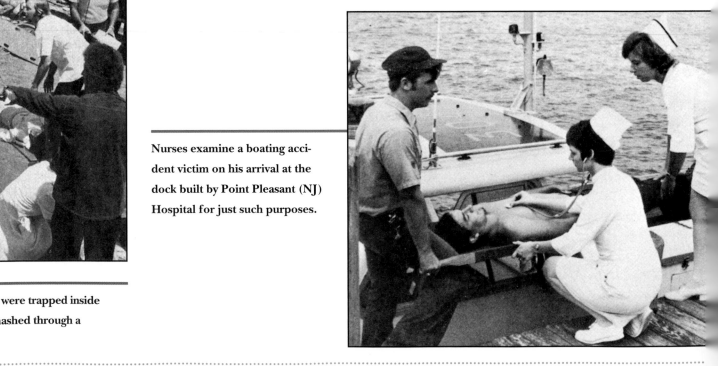

Nurses were there for students who were trapped inside an overturned school bus after it smashed through a California guardrail.

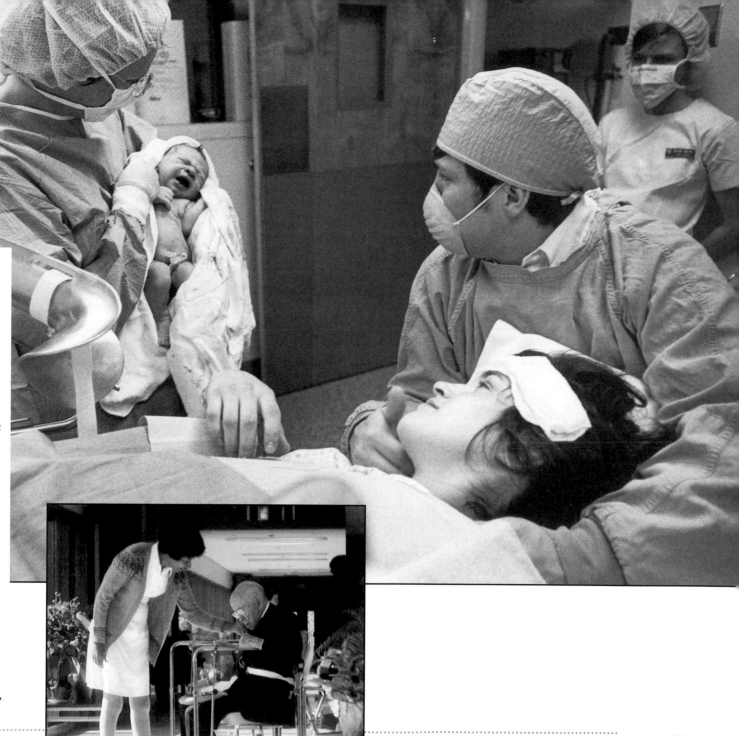

"*I was at a seminar for nursing directors and when I pleaded with them to please allow nurses to nurse, one got up and said, 'Do you mean to say that if a ward clerk is sick, you do not expect me to ask the staff nurses on that floor to do the ward clerk's chores?' I said that's exactly what I meant. But, I said, I'll make a compromise with you. On day one, you, as the director of nursing, tell the head nurse to go ahead and ask the staff nurses to take on the chores of the clerk, provided you promise me that if that ward clerk is still sick on day two, you will call the medical chief and say, 'Please send an intern to mind the telephone because the ward clerk is sick.' And on day three, will you ask the head of dietary 'to send a dietician to take on the job because the ward clerk is sick.' Then she finally realized the ridiculousness of the situation.*"

INGEBORG MAUKSCH,
OCTOBER 1975

In a high tech environment, just knowing the nurse is there can be reassuring to patients.

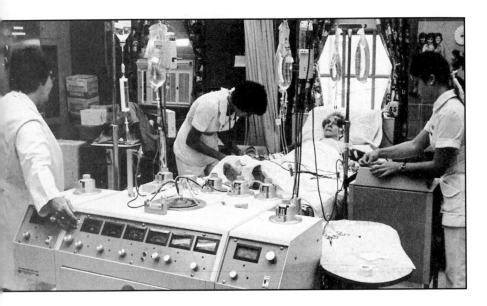

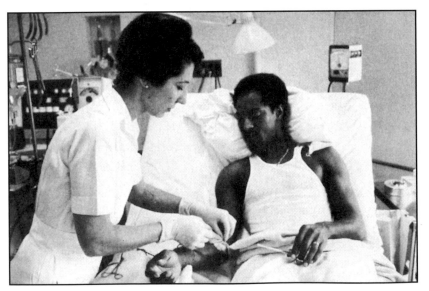

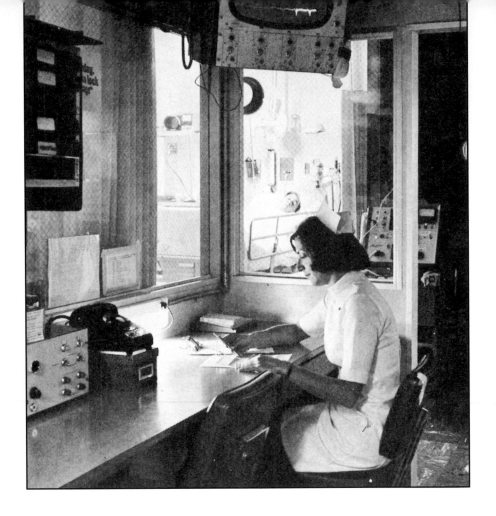

*T*he patients were then asked what they felt was the most positive aspect of their experience on the intensive care unit as well as the most negative. Thirteen responded that the most positive aspect was "knowing that the nurses were there every minute"; 10 answered simply, "nurses."

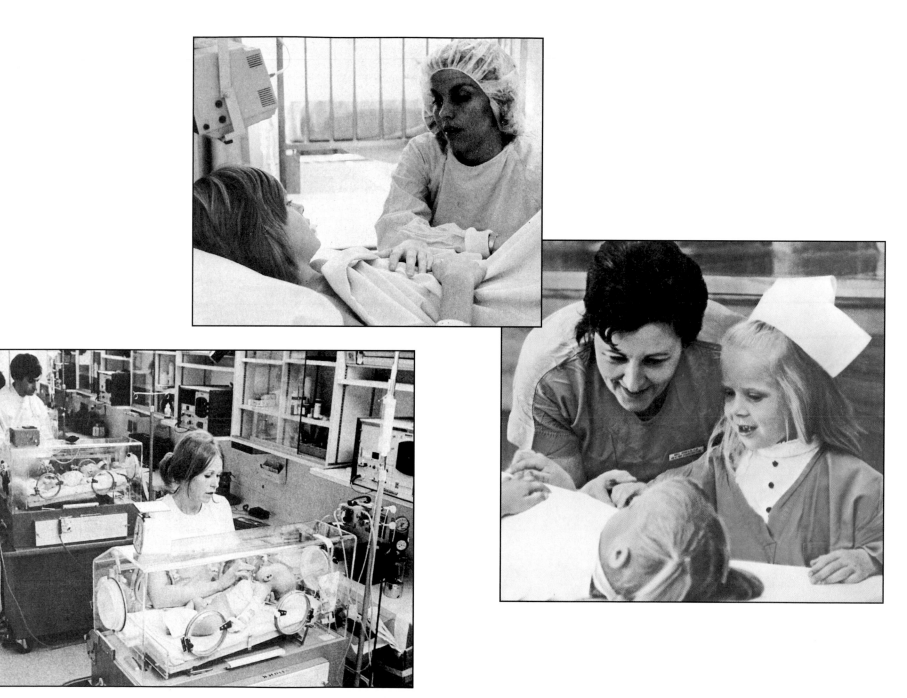

A Single Tear

I've really done it this time—
I've done what they've said not to—
  I'm emotionally involved.
Heaven knows I didn't want it to happen;
It just did.
  I had no control over it.

Her name came up on my assignment sheet
  And that started it.
I saw her lying there—each motion
  an effort,
Each breath proclaiming that it would be
  her last.
They said,
  "What a pity."
  "A terminal case."
  "She's so young."
And there I stood looking at this piece
  of humanity
And wondering what in God's name
  I could do.

There I was with what I felt constituted a
  strong will to live—
  My will to live was a mere drop in the
  bucket compared to hers
And what I did for her could never compare
  to what she's done for me.

So I began my day.
  I bathed her,
    Fluffed her pillows,
      Changed her position,
    Rubbed her back,
        Ran to the kitchen for Jello,
      or ginger ale,
      or ice cream.
  I took her temperature.
    I gave her medications.

I checked her oxygen,
  her I.V.,
    her catheter.
  I wiped her brow.
  I talked to her.
    I prayed with her.
      I prayed for her.

      Notes charted:
      Accurate Intake
        and Output;
    I.V. rate adjusted;
        Vital signs
      every two hours.

And all this time she lay there.
and she talked about the weather,
  the soon-coming spring,
  her home,
    her only grandchild she had seen
    for the first time at Christmas.

Her pulse now racing so fast I can't
  count it.
  Her urine is red.
    Her color is a blue-brown.
And yet she lay there
  Never smiling,
    But she never frowned.

Only once, after the priest had given her
  the Last Rites,
Did I see a single, solitary tear
  roll down her cheek.
And even though I counted her
  respirations,
And even though they were still
  the same,
  I could swear she breathed easier—
  for a time.
And so the day progressed.
  I watched, I waited, and God forgive me,
  I even hoped.

But always as I stood at the foot of her bed
She would open her eyes and say, "Hello."
I racked my brain to do something more.
  I put a drop of perfume behind each ear
  And brushed her hair.
  I got a sheepskin for her back.
  I put her get-well cards on the wall with
  masking tape
  So no one could complain that it would
  pull the paint off the wall.

I know very little about her personal
  history.
  (Why are charts so vague?)
And yet, if I were to judge what
  her task in life might be,
It would have to be
  Her faith, her perseverance, her
  unfailing clutch at life.

All this she has given to me:
  A shame for so little faith.
  A hope—for nothing is impossible,
  An acceptance of the inevitable.

She said, "Yes," to my offer for her
  narcotic.
And I plunged the needle into
  her pin-cushion buttocks.
She looked at me and asked,
  "Will you stay with me 'till it takes
  effect?"
"Of course," I smiled, "Just lie back and
  rest—I'll be right here."
  And I was.

I left a half hour later to finish some
  charting,
  Pour my afternoon meds,
  Check on other patients.

A buzzer rang and off I went.
It was a simple task and quickly completed,

A "thanks a lot" from him,
A "think nothing of it" from me.

I walked down the hall
  And another light flashed.
  Another simple task—and easily
  accomplished.

I walked down the hall to her room for
  another quick peek.
And in the doorway I stopped. . . .

I pushed the buzzer by her side.
  "Can I help you?" asked the speaker.
  "Send the head nurse in here, will you
  please?" I returned in a voice so calm
  it startled me.

Do you know what I thought about
  in those few minutes that I waited?
About the time my best-friend moved
  away, and when my dog died, and
  when our Lord said,
"Blessed are they which do hunger and
  thirst after righteousness:
  For they shall be filled."

I'm leaving the room now.
I've washed her face, brushed her hair,
  and changed her gown.
Evening shift said they'd watch for her
  husband and her teen-age daughter.

I'll go to the residence now and work on
  the bibliographies for class tomorrow,
  my care plan for Monday,
  the yearbook for next month's deadline.

I haven't cried yet, but I can feel it coming.
Perhaps tonight:
  in the solitude of my room. . . .

PEGGY DRINKWATER,
Methodist Hospital School of Nursing,
Philadelphia, Pennsylvania
JANUARY, 1971

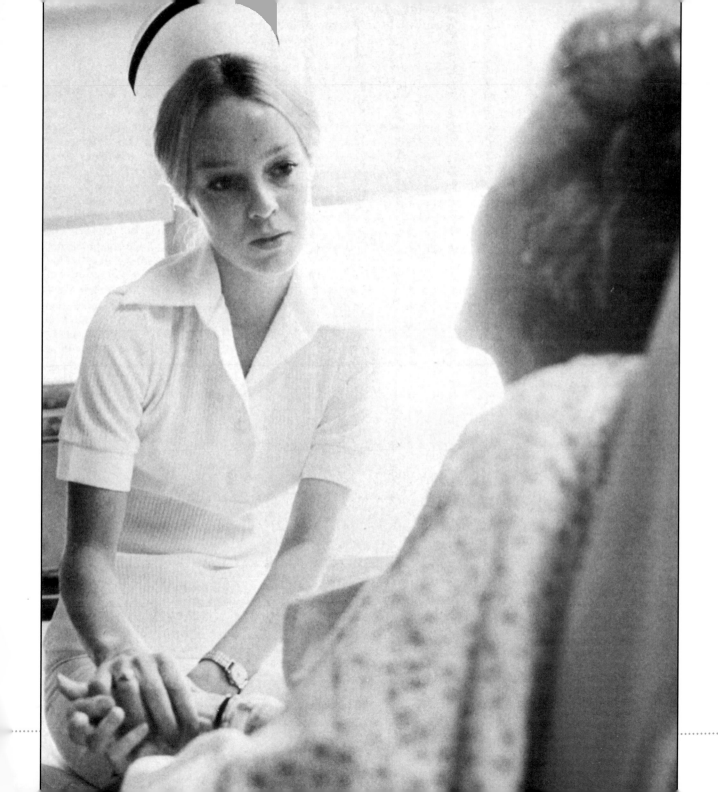

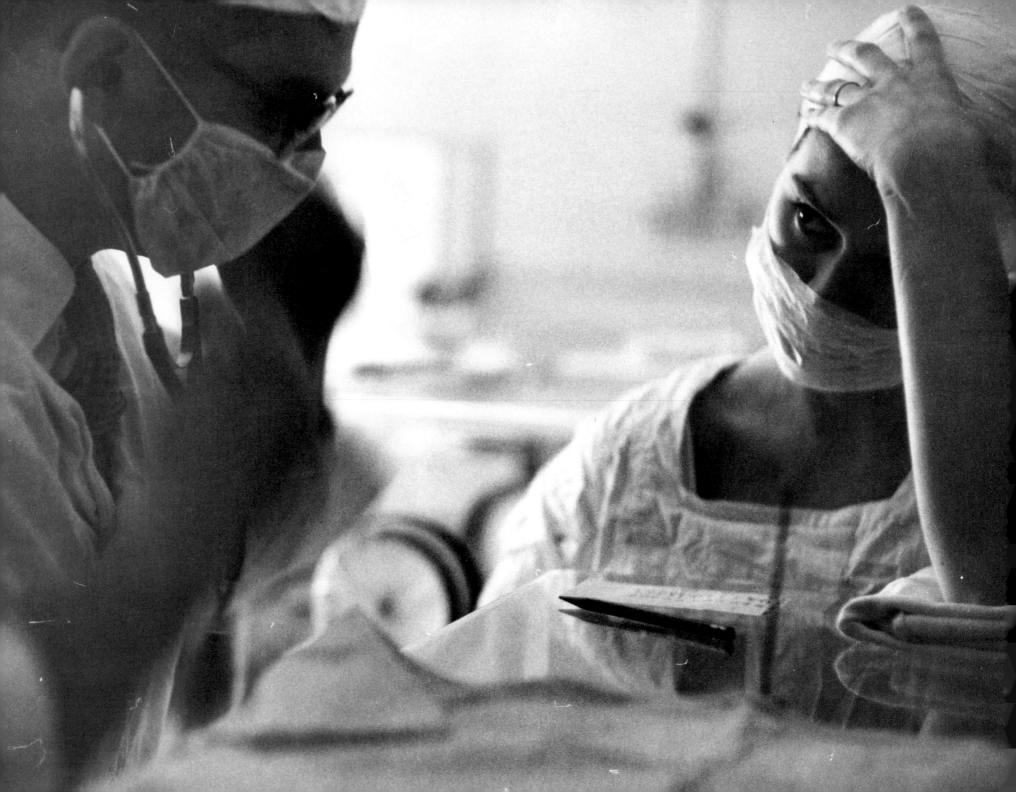

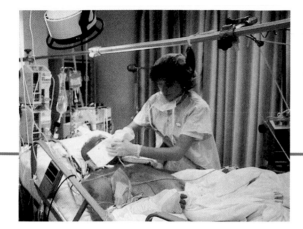

Redefining Practice

1980–1989

The cry of the 1980s throughout the country was nursing shortage. From the comfort of all-RN staffs and the satisfaction of primary nursing for patients and nurses alike, nurses moved into a familiar crisis—too few in number, in too great demand. Cost-cutting changes in health care also intensified, which deeply affected the profession.

Nurses were working long hours of overtime with acutely ill patients. Burnout often resulted when nurses felt isolated and powerless to effect change. Nurses wanted autonomy and control over their own practice, and more respect than they felt physicians showed them. Study after study—in Texas, New Jersey, Oregon, and Louisiana—showed that nurses were unhappy with the quality of care being given, the amount of non-nursing work they were expected to do, and the lack of administrative support. Many would leave and go to work for supplemental staffing agencies where they had control, at least, over their working hours. Others became entrepreneurs, setting up their own staffing agencies or nursing centers. Hospitals responded by trying to add more staff. Bonuses and bounties were offered to anyone who could bring in more nurses.

Research and experimentation in education were providing, if not answers to job dissatisfaction, at least a place to start. The unification model of nursing—a three-pronged effort involving collaboration in service, education, and research—was put in place at Case Western Reserve in Cleveland, at the University of Rochester Medical Center, at Rush-Presbyterian-St. Luke's Medical Center in Chicago, and at the University of Florida in Gainesville. In other places, strands of unification like faculty involvement in patient care, faculty appointments for service personnel, and joint appointments were proliferating. Clinical ladders were also being instituted to provide staff nurses the opportunity for planned career development.

The nurse practitioner (NP) movement also flourished throughout the 1980s, but the NPs' inability to get reimbursement from third-party payers like Medicare and insurance companies continued to hamper their efforts. Moreover, they sought prescriptive authority, which meant they needed political presence. N-CAP, the American Nurses Association's political arm, was providing that presence, working for the election of state and federal legislators who would support nursing's causes.

Toward the end of the 1980s, the American Medical Association announced its answer to the nursing shortage. It would set up nine-month programs to prepare "Registered Care Technologists (RCTs)," a proposal that incensed and unified nurses. As a result of nursing's opposition, the RCT proposal came to naught. Although one pilot program was started, the students never completed their training.

Concern about health care costs was mounting in the 1980s and the use of diagnosis-related groups (DRGs) to cap hospital reimbursement spread from the federal government, which had developed them to contain Medicare costs, to private insurers as well. By the end of the decade, hospitals were closing wards and establishing short-stay day and ambulatory units, and nurses were moving from inpatient to outpatient settings.

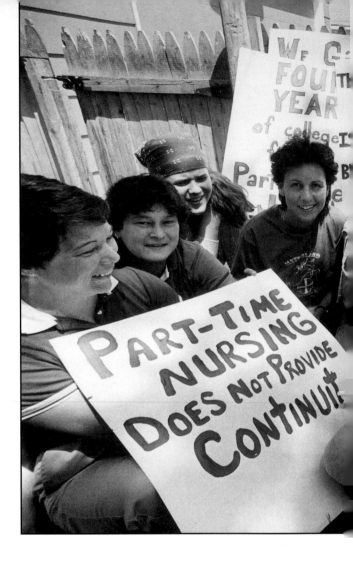

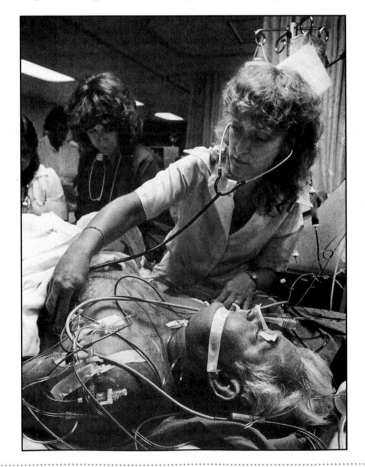

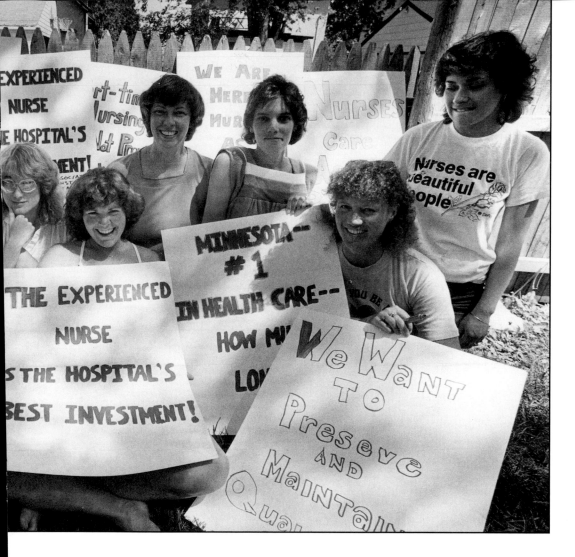

Letters

"I'm tired . . ."

I look at the position ads and, frankly, I'm tired of "having a heart" and "accepting a challenge." My heart has been broken too many times and challenges have become depressing. What will arouse me is a salary of $35,000 a year. Any takers?

May 1981

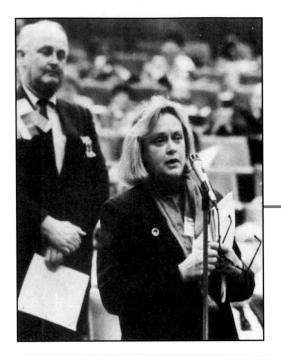

Budget cuts and declining enrollments took their toll on nursing schools from coast to coast, with UCLA, Skidmore, and Boston University closing their undergraduate programs.

"There is no compromise on the RCT issue," said ANA's president Lucille Joel at an AMA meeting. Nurses nationwide united and spoke out against those who would replace nurses at the bedside with non-nurse caregivers.

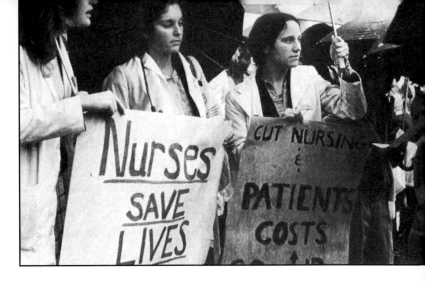

UCLA students lead a rainy-day march to protest proposals to close the undergraduate program.

In all weather, RNs battled for better staffing.

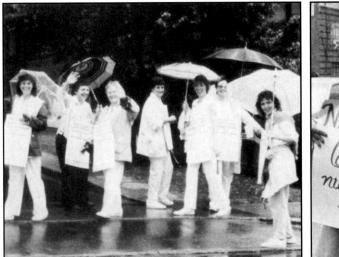

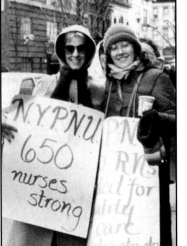

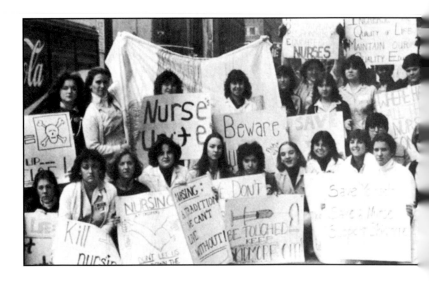

Students show a united front against a vote to close Skidmore's school of nursing.

Nursing had many influential supporters . . .

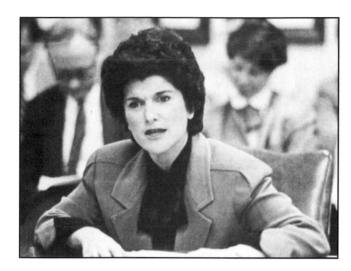

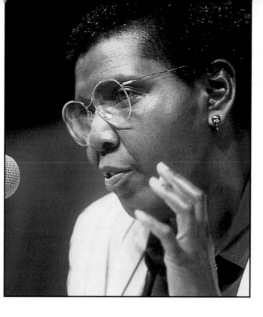

"This is no time for nurses' numbers to be declining: Congress has just expanded Medicare. Without nurses we don't have a system."

BARBARA JORDAN

Luci Baines Johnson, daughter of the late President Lyndon Johnson, told a Congressional committee that cutting nursing programs would be an exercise in "false economy" since nurses provide the most cost-effective care.

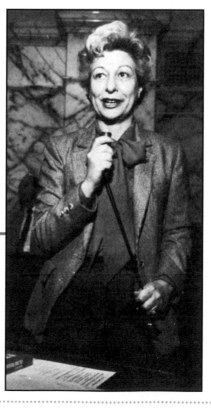

Maryland legislator Marilyn Goldwater, RN, argued for a state commission to study nursing issues. The bill passed.

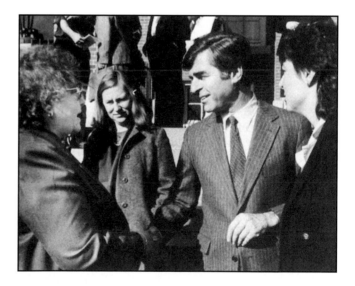

and Massachusetts Governor Michael Dukakis offered his support.

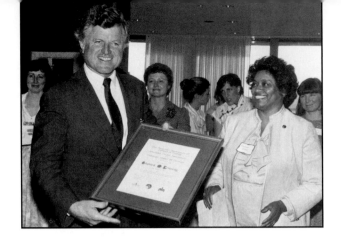

Senator Edward Kennedy (D-Mass.) accepts a plaque from ANA President Barbara Nichols for his support.

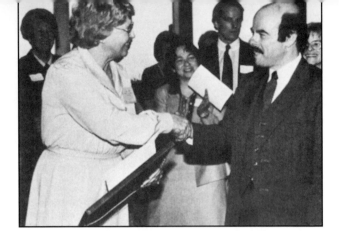

AACN President Billye Brown presents a citation to Representative Henry Waxman (D-Calif.).

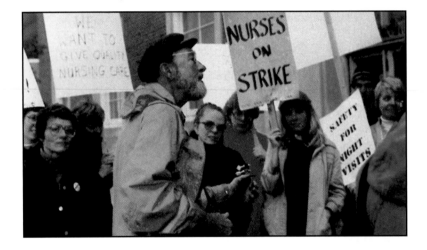

From celebrities like Pete Seeger to senior citizens, support came from all sides.

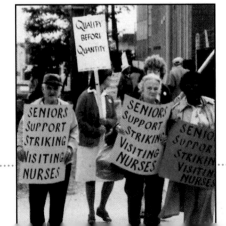

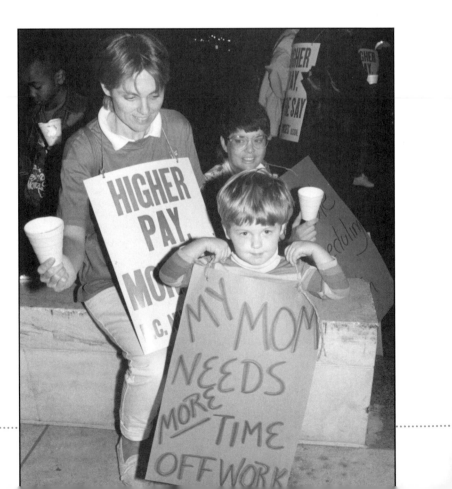

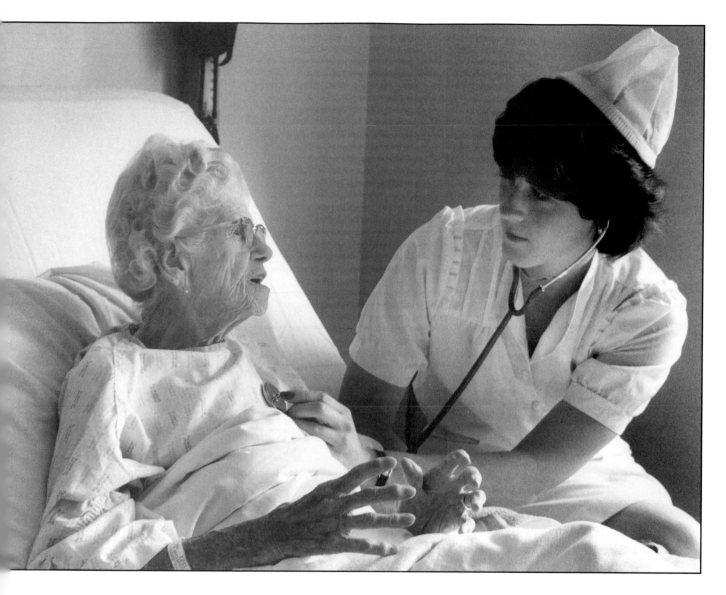

"*I wanted to tell the world that the person in this bed was not always like this. She'd ranked first in her high-school class, raised six children, worked, took care of my dying father, and traveled all over the world. I wanted to shout, "That woman in there—the one you can't understand—she's not what you see."*

MARCH 1988

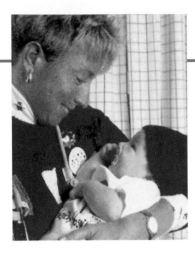

Commentary

Patricia Benner

Caring Practices

Caring practices have more than sentiment attached to them, they are laden with knowledge and relational skill—the abilities that allow us to respond to another's personhood and plight. Caring practices both forge and tap our common humanity. Caring practices in times of illness and vulnerability, conditions all finite embodied beings share, are life saving and life enhancing.

Often the most effective caregiving work remains hidden in the name of preserving the identity, independence, and integrity of the other. These are the gossamer strands of caring for the other that weave us together and open new possibilities. New steps are taken and new identities forged on these relational highways.

Comforting another is relational. Comfort measures are offered. It is the other who receives and elaborates them into support, help, and strength. Some human suffering is beyond comfort, so that one can only offer. Nurses live with the ethical tension of providing adequate pain medication and sedation, while not substituting these numbing remedies for human solace and comfort. This tension is central in the care of critically ill infants who must learn to be comforted by other human beings, through being held, positioned, and nurtured by comforting human touch, soothing voice, and song. As Nightingale taught, technical interventions are usually temporary stopgap measures to be used until the body is healed and regains its own ways.

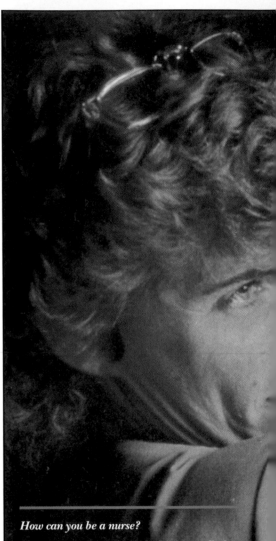

How can you be a nurse?
How can you bear to watch children suffer?
Wait until you've rocked and soothed a suffering child into peaceful sleep, and you feel the child's relief washing over you like a blessing. Then you won't need to ask.

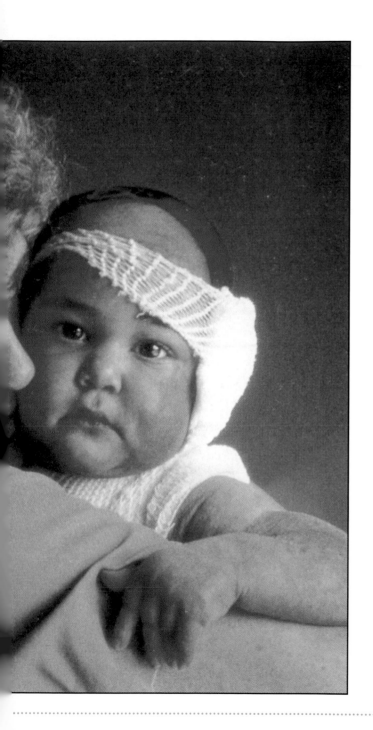

In critical care units where life is fragile, caregiving practices render alien environments and heroic technical interventions safe. Nurses talk of knowing the patient and family, of following the body's lead, of comforting relationships, of wooing patients back into their own life worlds by familiar sights and sounds. Without these caring practices, our highly technical interventions would be too alien, too frightening, and too painful to endure.

Sometimes the ethics of care and justice are pitted against one another as if one is more important than the other. We need more justice in our caregiving work, and more care in our systems of justice. In times of vulnerability and breakdown, justice will not be sufficient; care, mercy and generosity are needed. Yet when justice is absent, acts of care are required for survival and hope until justice can be achieved.

When care is reduced to feelings and attitudes only, then caregiving work is trivialized or sentimentalized. Sentiment is necessary to perceive the plight of others and the need for action, but on its own, it is not sufficient. One must school one's practical abilities to respond to suffering, need, and vulnerability through developing ways of helping and relating.

Biological birthing is only the beginning. Social birthing requires ongoing labors of care. The society that ignores this central fact does so at its own peril.

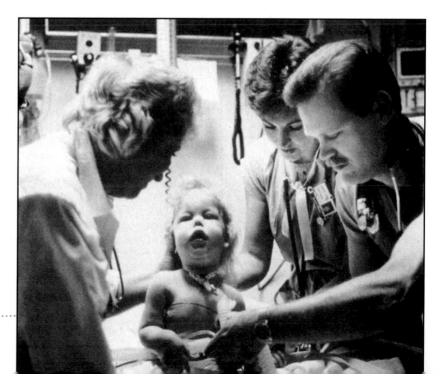

How can you be a nurse? So many of your patients are so old, so sick, these days. How can you bear the thought that, in the end, your care may make no difference?

Wait until you've used your hands and eyes and voice to dispel terror, to show a helpless person that his life is respected, that he has dignity. Your caring helps him care about himself . . .

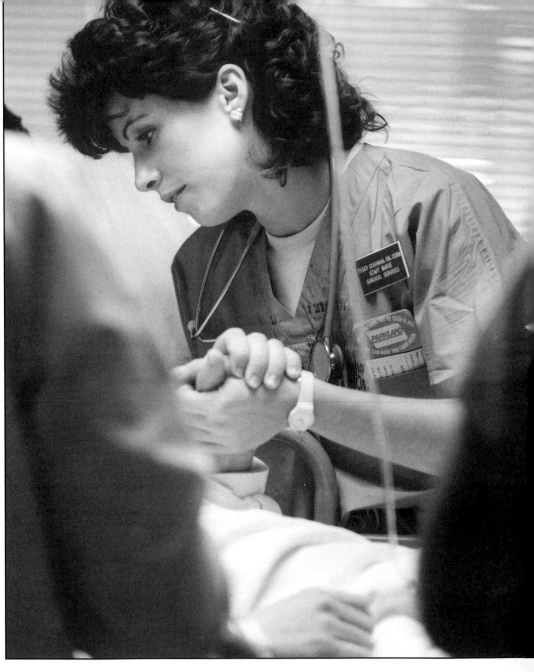

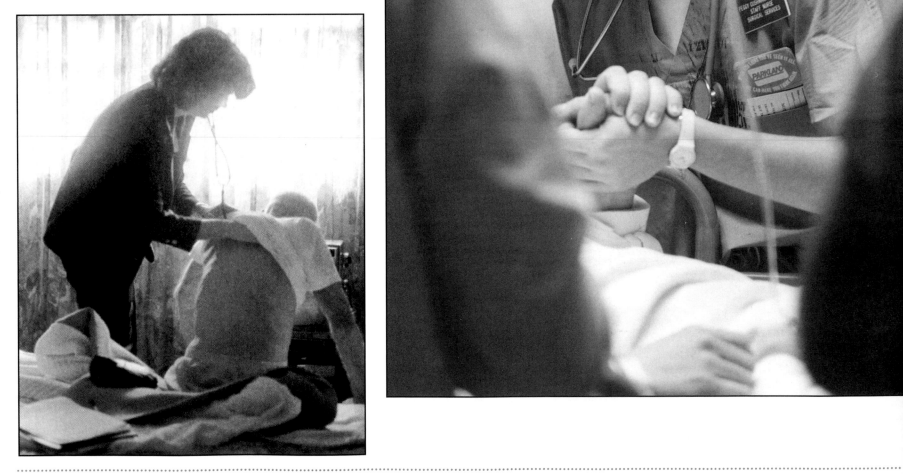

How can you be a nurse? How can you bear the sight and smell of feces?

Wait until you've been anxious about the diarrhea that nothing has stopped in an AIDS patient. Finally, your strategies work and you see and smell normal stool. You'll welcome that smell . . .

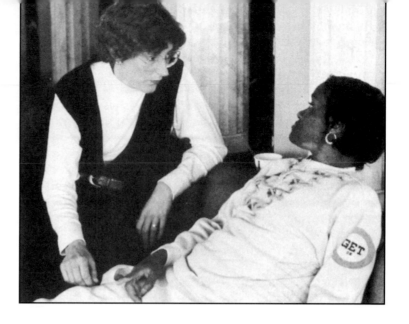

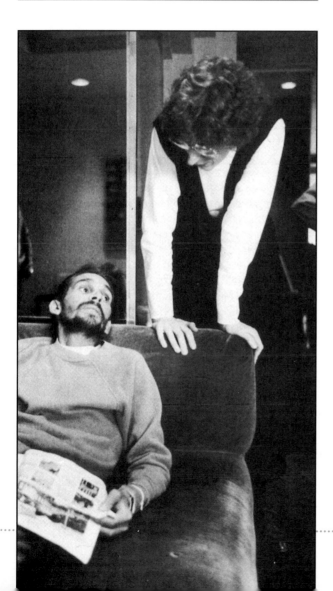

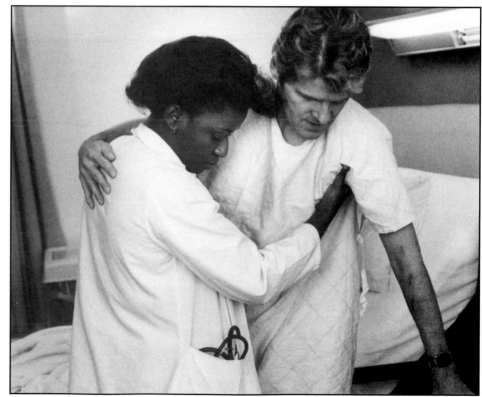

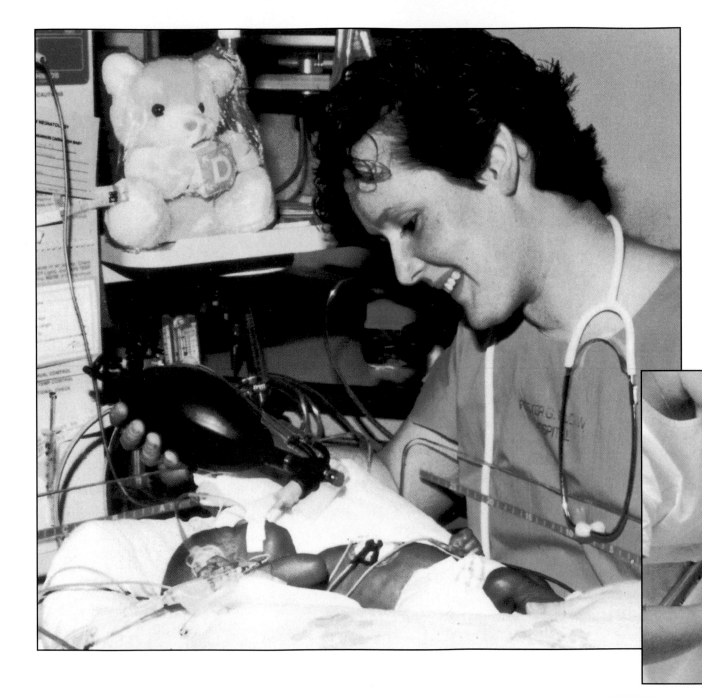

How can you be a nurse? How can you bear the sound of babies crying? Wait until your combination of vigilance, bulldog advocacy, and gentle handling has given a preemie's lungs the time they needed to develop, and you hear his first lusty cry. You'll laugh out loud!

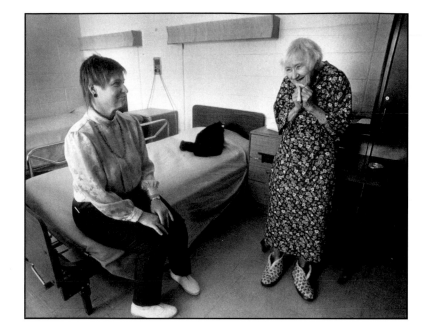

How can you be a nurse? How can you bear to care for frustrating, confused Alzheimer's patients?

Wait until you've devised a combination of strategies that provide exercise and permit safe wandering, and you see a lift, almost a spring, in a patient's shuffling gait. You'll feel the lightness of Baryshnikov in your own step that day.

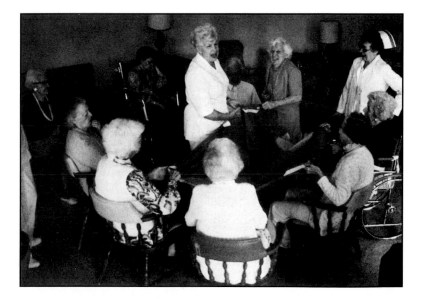

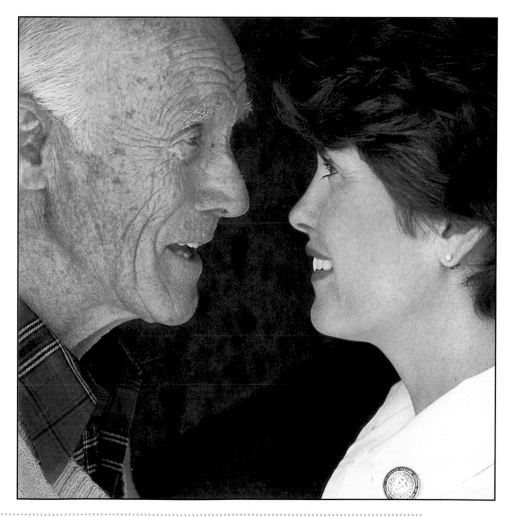

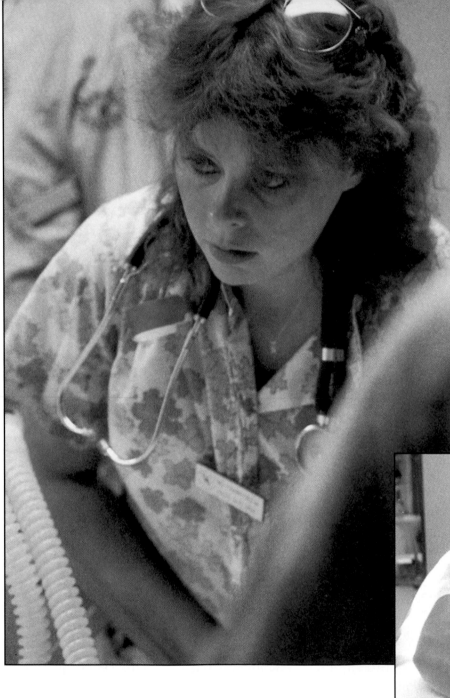

So you keep choosing to be a nurse. You have days of frustration, nights of despair, terrible angers. Your highs and lows are peaks and chasms, not hills and valleys. The defeats come more than often enough to keep you humble: the problems you can't untangle, the lives that seep away too fast, the meanings that elude your understanding.

But you keep working at it, learning from it, knowing the next peak lies ahead.

MARY MALLISON
EDITORIAL, APRIL 1987

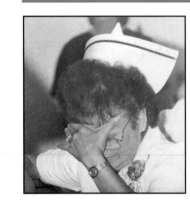

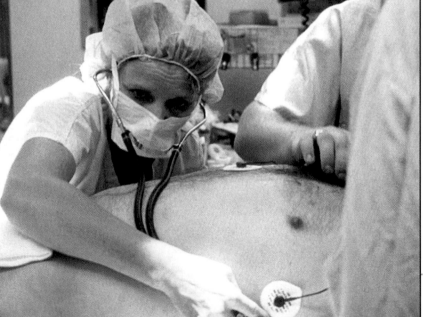

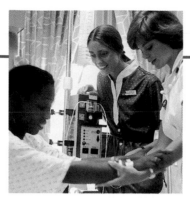

Commentary

Ada Sue Hinshaw

Nursing Research and the Explosion of Knowledge

Nursing research experienced rapid growth during the 1980s. This expansion occurred primarily because nursing scientists focused on generating knowledge for the practice of the profession and because of the dramatic increase in the resources available to support such important work.

In the late 1980s, several nursing scholars suggested that nursing research needed to be firmly focused on the substantive information required to guide practice rather than on philosophical and methodological dilemmas of scientific inquiry. The creation of the National Center for Nursing Research (NCNR) in 1985 at the National Institutes of Health (NIH) moved the support of the discipline's research programs into the mainstream of health science. As a result, nursing research has advanced dramatically.

The establishment of the NCNR, now the National Institute of Nursing Research (NINR), brought with it an increase in federal resources for nursing research and research training. Even more importantly, the creation of the NINR at the NIH became a visible symbol of the federal legitimization of nursing research as a field of study worthy of national support and recognition.

Such rapid growth in nursing research was made possible because major foundations had been built with the support of the Division of Nursing (DN) of the Health Resources and Services Agency (HRSA) of the Department of Health and Human Services (DHHS). Federal support for nursing research began in 1955 with the creation of the Research Grants and Fellowship Branch within the Division of Nursing Resources, originally established at the NIH in the Bureau of Medical Services. The Division of Nursing systematically offered a series of federal programs that built the infrastructure that supported the expansion of nursing research in the 1990s.

In the 1980s, three programs funded the research training of nurses: the Special Predoctoral and Postdoctoral Research Fellowships, the Nurse Scientist Graduate Training program, and the individual National Research Service Award program. These programs were established to prepare a cadre of nurse scientists who could build research programs in university schools of nursing, develop doctoral programs with a nursing major, and conduct sophisticated research. Two other programs were aimed at developing faculty research and research centers within schools of nursing. An additional program was focused on enhancing developing doctoral programs. This federal support was provided over a period of three decades. The programs began in 1955 with $625,000 allocated for nursing research and training for that year, and ultimately reached an annual amount between $3 million and $5 million.

Professional support for nursing research was also critical in the creation of the NINR. The strong leadership of the Tri-Council members (ANA, American Association of Colleges of Nursing, NLN, and the American Organization of Nurse Executives), using their legislative offices, organizational networks, and political savvy, as well as the support of the nursing scientific community, was a major force in establishing the National Center for Nursing Research (NCNR) through the Health Research Extension Act of 1985.

With the establishment of the NCNR, increased federal resources were allocated to nursing research, which provided a strong surge of energy to the generation of knowledge for nursing practice. The initial budget of $16.5 million in 1986 grew to $63.5 million by 1998. Although this was a sizable increase, the amount is limited given the staggering research opportunities and the crucial need for information to guide nursing and health care.

A series of NCNR major initiatives provided guidance for scientific development. These initiatives focused resources on primary areas of study, which included setting national nursing research priorities (National Nursing Research Agenda), developing a trajectory for research training and career development, increasing interdisciplinary research, and promoting international research endeavors. Priorities were selected based on how critical a

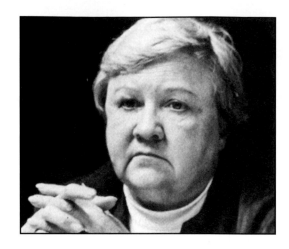

Among the pioneers in nursing research, Susan Gortner (below) chief, Nursing Research Branch, Division of Nursing, and Phyllis Verhonick, (above) director of research at the University of Virginia School of Nursing.

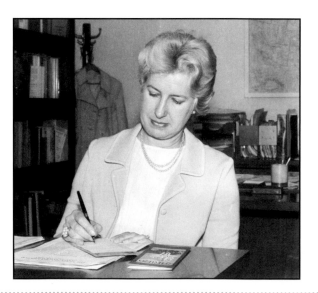

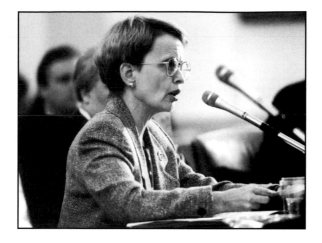

Strong leadership from nursing organizations, particularly ANA, NLN, AACN, and AONE, was a major force in establishing the National Institute of Nursing Research. Here, Barbara Redman testifies.

given clinical problem or issue was to the health of the public, the ability of nursing as a profession to influence it, and the availability of nurse investigators to study it. In research training, the emphasis was on postdoctoral study and midcareer development, since the lack of resources had prevented the development of a research career for many nurses.

Moving nursing research into the NIH enhanced the interdisciplinary possibilities for collaborative investigation. Also, the globalization of nursing research through the international initiative linked the NCNR with the International Council of Nurses and Sigma Theta Tau International. Each of these moves broadened the opportunities for nurse researchers in generating knowledge.

The NCNR was redesignated the National Institute of Nursing Research (NINR) in June of 1993. The professional nursing community, through the Tri-Council, initiated legislation for the redesign. Concurrently, the NIH, through the Director, Dr. Bernadine Healy, requested redesignation to institute status by way of the executive branch of the DHHS. No additional funds were requested. The NCNR was functioning as an institute with a similar legislative mandate and a full set of programs consistent with those of the other NIH institutes.

Exciting outcomes are evident from the rapid growth in nursing research during the 1990s. Multiple research programs focus on important health issues, such as health promotion across the life span. Sample investigative areas include culturally specific prevention interventions for low-birth-weight infants; promoting healthy lifestyle decisions for adolescents; decision making processes for estrogen replacement therapy for midlife women; exercise benefits for the older individual; and symptom assessment and management of clinical problems such as pain, fatigue, urinary incontinence, and wandering behavior in the elderly. Restructuring health care with a focus on balancing quality and cost outcomes is also an ongoing area of investigation.

Nursing research is beginning to inform health care policy through federal commissions and agency programs. The continuing pool of scientists depends on stronger research training programs with an emphasis on earlier entry into the research trajectory. A major challenge for the future is to enhance the ability of nursing research to shape and inform health policy at multiple levels. There is a need to conceptualize the relationship of research to policy and to develop explicit strategies for enhancing it.

Dana Delaney, who portrayed Vietnam nurse Colleen McMurphy in the television drama, "China Beach," was one of the celebrities who participated in nurse recruitment drives in the 1980s.

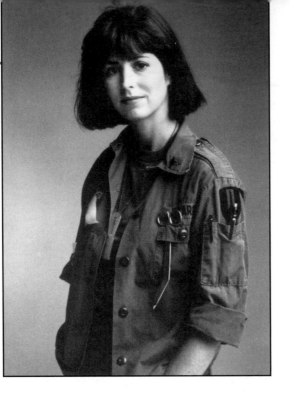

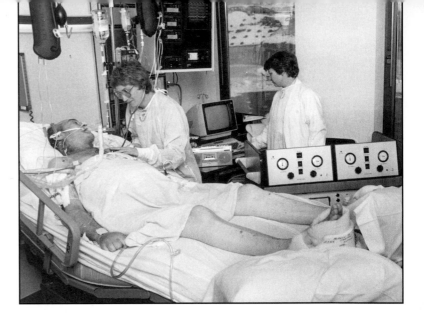

The intense nursing care needed by Barney Clark, first recipient of an artificial heart, received worldwide publicity.

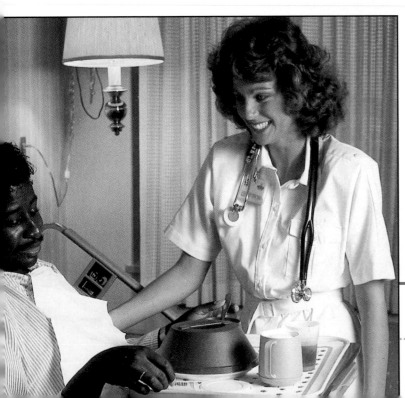

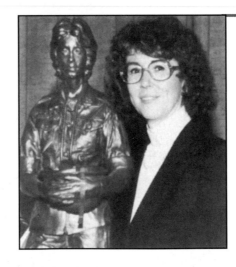

Donna-Marie Boulay, chair of the Vietnam Women's Memorial Project, next to the statue the group wanted erected to commemorate the 11,000 women veterans who served in Vietnam. Boulay and Diane Carlson Evans, both nurses who served in Vietnam, spearheaded the drive that erupted into a battle when the federal Fine Arts Commission refused to approve the statue. Congressional support, however, later pushed approval through for a different monument.

Kaye Lani Rae, RN, Miss America 1988, toured the country visiting hospitals and garnering favorable publicity for nursing.

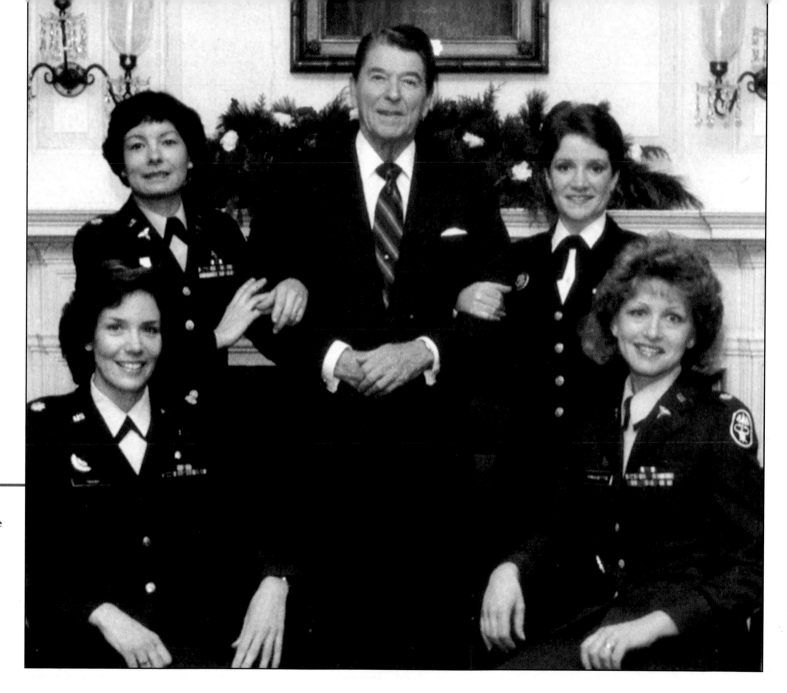

Four of America's finest—
the Armed Forces nominate
their best emergency and
ICU specialists for White
House positions—pose in
uniform with their former
Commander-in-Chief and
primary patient.

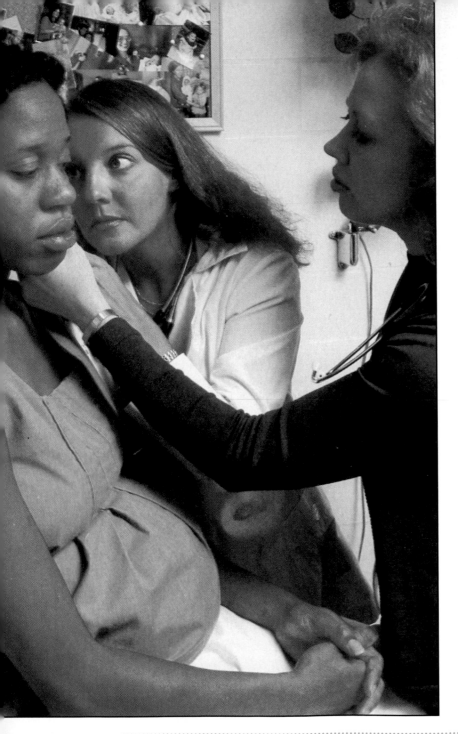

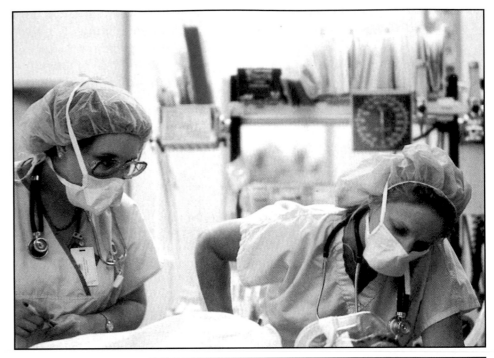

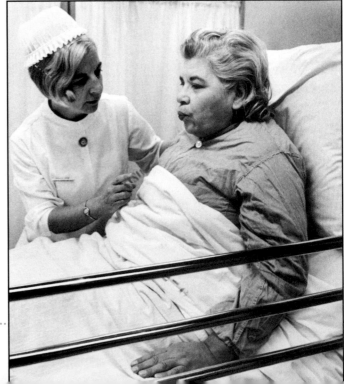

Caring is the candle that lights the dark, that permits us to find answers where others see none.

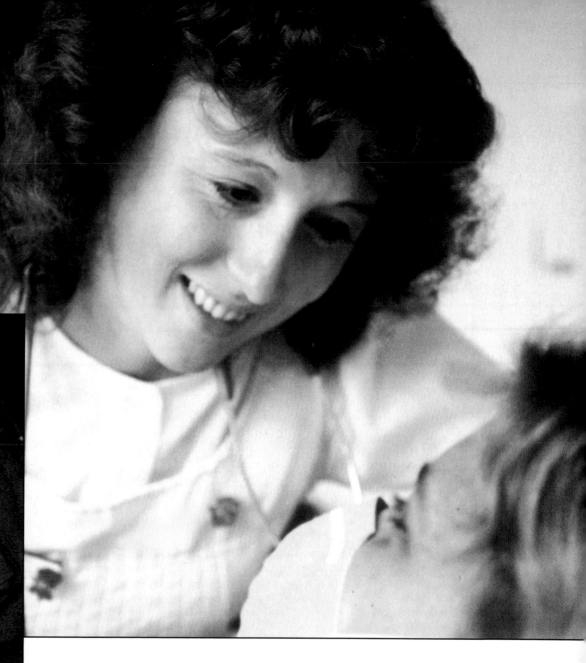

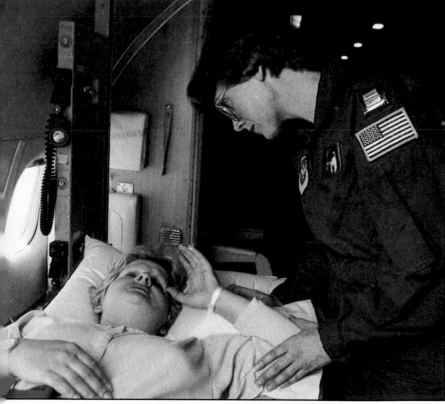

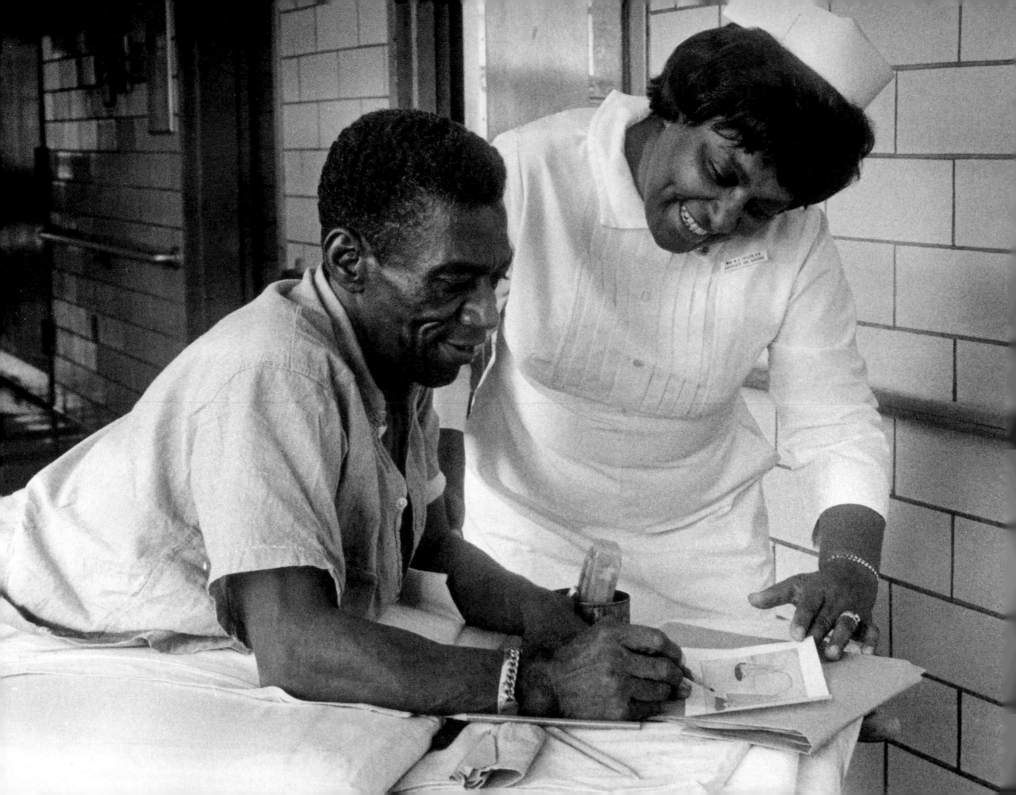

It helps to remember the patient's struggle as well as his strength, his fight as well as his acceptance, and his fear as well as his serenity.

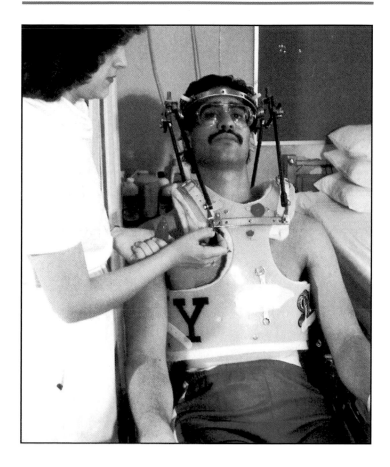

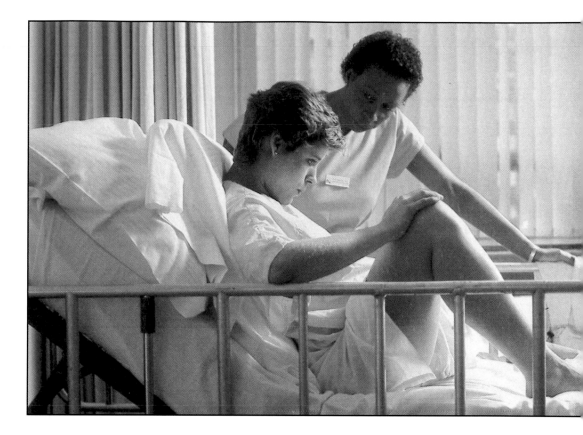

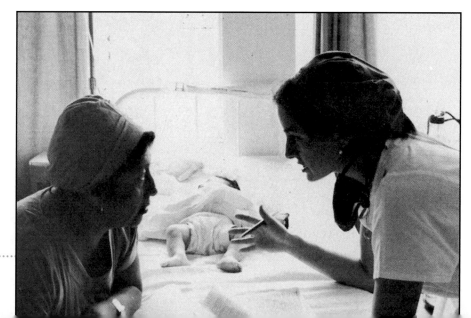

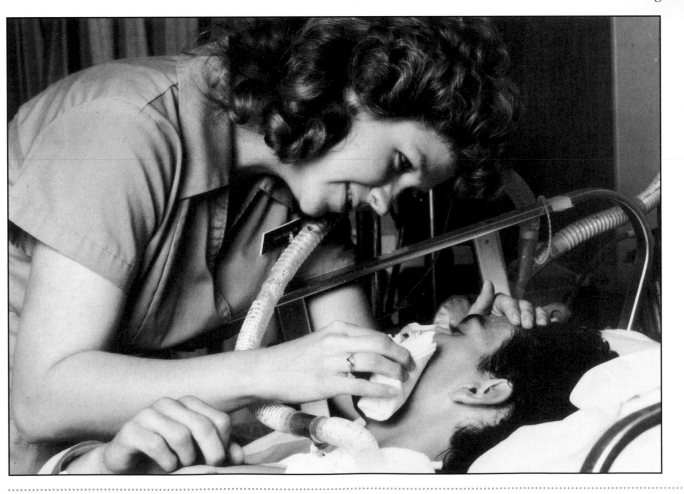

*"**N**urses have always pushed, pulled, and coached patients through their illnesses. Nurses have always made the technology bearable and understandable, have known when to use it more frequently or when to gradually withdraw it. Whether the technology is poultices or ventilators, the nursing attitudes are the same."*

MARY MALLISON
EDITORIAL, MARCH 1988

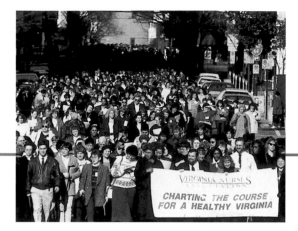

CHARTING THE COURSE FOR A HEALTHY VIRGINIA

The Nineties: Anticipating the New Millennium

The 1990s have placed nurses in a tumultuous health care environment. The decade began with some halcyon times—more and more hospitals were going to all-RN staffs; a swelling number of institutions were adopting primary nursing as their nursing philosophy; student enrollments had increased; and research confirmed that higher levels of RN staffing were associated with lower mortality and fewer complications. Overall, nurses felt more appreciated, both psychologically and financially.

At the start of the 1990s, the emphasis was on cost effectiveness, and nurses believed they upheld this objective. The American Nurses Association (ANA) and the National League for Nursing (NLN) enthusiastically hammered out *Nursing's Agenda for Health Care Reform,* which 60 nursing organizations had signed on to, and which proposed much of what would be in the Clinton Administration's health care program. Although Congress voted down that program, many of its elements—like managed care and health maintenance organizations—were put into place, but without the safeguards that might have protected the poor, the uninsured, and ultimately, everyone else. The operative phrase became "cost containment," and hospitals began to downsize, to merge, to substitute unlicensed assistive personnel for RNs, and to limit lengths of stay until legislation forced minimum stays for mothers and newborns and a 48-hour minimum postmastectomy.

Despite these disappointments in the health care system, there have been some bright spots. There are still magnet hospitals, so deemed for their good patient care by the American Nurses Credentialing Center, which emphasize the quality of their nurses in marketing campaigns that educate the public and benefit the profession. Also, many nurses who were forced out of hospitals are finding satisfying careers in home health and other community-based settings. Nurse-managed clinics—once the refuge of the rural poor—are now gaining regard and acceptance across economic and geographic lines. In addition, a three-year Medicare demonstration project, funded by the Health Care Financing Administration, is testing a nurse-managed ambulatory care program at four sites: Carondelet Health Care in Tucson, Arizona; Carle Clinic Association in Urbana, Illinois; the Visiting Nurse Service of New York, New York and the Living at Home/Block Nursing Program in St. Paul, Minnesota.

During the 1990s, enormous enthusiasm has been engendered for the roles of advanced practice nurses who have proved their mettle in primary care and acute care settings and in tertiary settings as well. They bring a unique perspective to traditional health care; many of them support holistic and complementary therapies and teach healthy lifestyle practices.

As the decade draws to a close, cost containment has seemingly become a way of life in health care management. In addition, rumblings of a new nursing shortage are being heard. Once again comes the realization that substitute personnel cannot safely replace skilled nurses. And so, once again, the cycle begins.

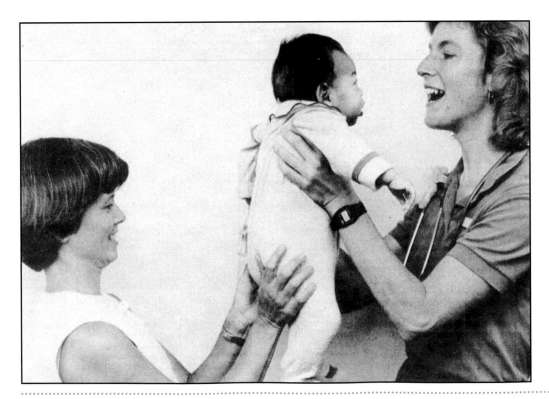

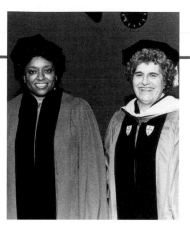

Commentary

Margretta Madden Styles

The New Wave of Credentialing

Credentialing encompasses the means—governmental and nongovernmental, mandatory and voluntary— whereby nurses and nursing programs and services are regulated. Licensing, certification, and accreditation credentials are awarded for meeting or exceeding established performance standards. Political, technological, and health care forces have dramatically changed credentialing philosophies and practices.

Telecommunications and geopolitical alignments, such as the European Union and the North American Free Trade Alliance, are rendering obsolete the concept of "jurisdiction" as the centerpiece of regulation. International trade agreements mandate free movement of services as well as goods. Professionals must be able to engage in cross-border practice by physical or virtual travel. "Telehealth" and "telenursing" are changing the very definitions of "caring." Within the United States, mutual recognition compacts are developing among states, and talk of national licensure fills the air.

Powerful American sentiments of deregulation, decentralization, privatization, and competition are sweeping other continents, creating gaps in government protection; disaffection, insecurity, and restiveness among consumers; and opportunities for voluntary forms of credentialing to fill the void. The health care industry has been the cauldron within which these forces have bubbled most vigorously because of the unprecedented science- and technology-driven advances in practice and the economically driven restructuring of the delivery system. Incompetence among health care professionals who can't or don't keep up, systems pressing for cost reductions, and monitoring by resource-starved and bureaucratically strangled licensing bodies have proven to be a fatal combination for some consumers, a combination that fortunately has given rise to changes characterizing the late twentieth-century credentialing movement.

Continuous quality improvement has become the banner of the day, and the emphasis is now on partnerships between the government, providers, professionals, and consumers. Nursing, with its long tradition of patient advocacy, is very active at the center of many of those partnerships. In this environment, advanced practice nursing has gained increasing popularity.

Advanced practice nursing is recognized as highly valuable for a number of reasons. Nurses with advanced education, expanded practice privileges, and greater autonomy increase the availability of primary health care to underserved populations—care that is demonstrably of good quality yet costs less. The spread of advanced practice nursing, however, has forced a reexamination of the systems for credentialing nurses to ensure that special competence is maintained within the cadre of more institutionally independent practitioners.

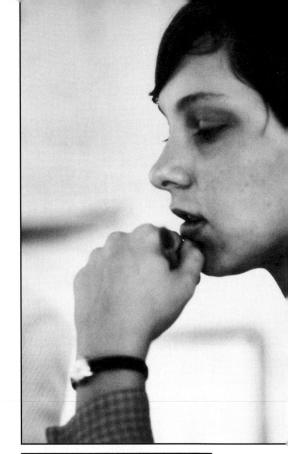

In the 1990s, a partnership was forged between mandatory state licensure authorities, which set practice standards at the level of entering associate degree graduates, and national, nongovernmental bodies that certify graduate-prepared specialists. The national bodies submitted to external, expert scrutiny to ensure that their credentials were acceptable for regulatory purposes and were, in turn, recognized by most of the state boards. These national certifying agencies are intensely engaged in improving methods for determining the continuing competence of certified nurses practicing within the swift currents of health care change.

The consumer voice in the partnership is heard via collaboration with advocacy organizations and the increasing appointment of public members to licensing, certifying, and accreditation boards. Voluntary credentialing bodies recognize that if they are to serve effectively, they must engage in active public information campaigns to inform consumers about their health care choices.

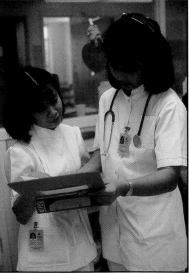

The goal of organizations providing health care services is to provide high-quality care in an efficient manner and to be acknowledged as a good choice for consumers. American voluntary accreditation bodies, such as the Joint Commission on Accreditation of Health Care Organizations, have long

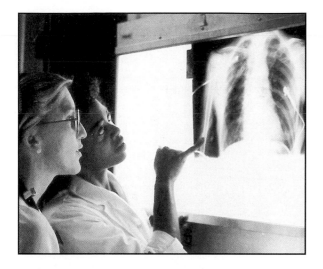

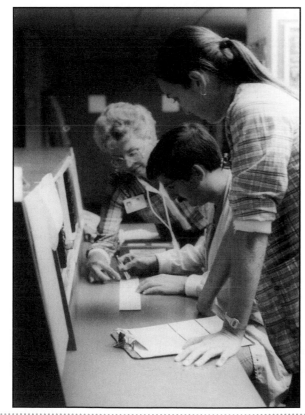

served as a surrogate for governmental regulation prevailing elsewhere in the world. Such accreditation ensures that minimum standards have been met and maintained throughout the institution or system.

Within the fast-moving scenario of late twentieth century health care, nursing, more than most professions, has the public trust, an asset to be invested wisely. This has afforded a new opportunity for nurses to excel and serve as consumer partners. Professional bodies, such as the American Nurses Credentialing Center, can survey and single out exceptional nursing services in hospital or community settings for special recognition, setting forth demonstrated indicators of high-quality nursing care. Institutions also benefit from this process, by improving their services to meet these high standards and being recognized for this achievement.

Every sector, every stakeholder stands to gain from mutual commitment and collaborative endeavor in setting and applying standards for nurses and nursing services. A comprehensive, multifaceted credentialing system can, in fact, serve as an advocate for nurses and their career enhancement, as a tool for involving and informing consumers, as an edge for health care systems competing for quality and consumers, and as a value indicator for public and private payers.

Credentialing deserves to be celebrated in this century of caring. And it promises an even greater contribution in the next.

Marching in Washington, RNs Warn Against Cuts in Care

*W*ASHINGTON, DC—"It's our Woodstock," an RN explained to reporters as nurses by the thousand rallied here and marched the length of Pennsylvania Avenue, chanting "Save nurses, save lives."

MAY 1995

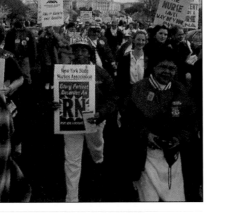

Thousands of nurses came from every state to join in the March on Washington on March 31, 1995.

Early in the '90s, nursing unveiled its own plan for reforming the nation's ailing health care system and "took it on the road." *Nursing's Agenda for Health Care Reform* was supported by 60 nursing organizations.

ANA President Lucille Joel explains nursing's consensus plan for reform to Arkansas Governor Bill Clinton in 1991.

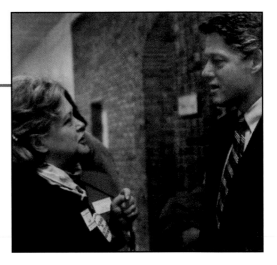

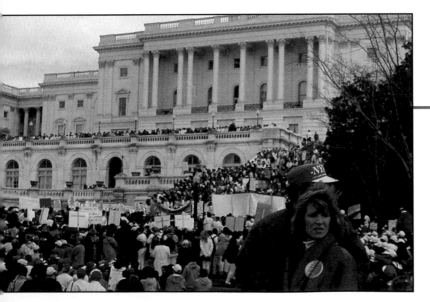

Rallying at the Capitol's west front, marchers were urged to "fight back" and "save lives."

"*W*e must not—we cannot—tolerate or adapt to a system that puts the interests of employers before the needs of patients. We must resist every hospital restructuring move and every work reorganization scheme that puts business decisions ahead of caregiving ones."

—JOURNALIST SUZANNE GORDON IN A SPEECH TO THE NURSES' RALLY AT THE CAPITOL ON MARCH 31, 1995.

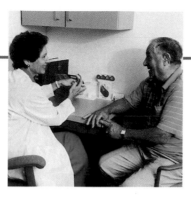

Commentary

*Mary Mundinger
and Nancy Boccuzzi*

Breaking Boundaries in Advanced Nursing Practice

Columbia Advanced Practice Nurse Associates (CAPNA), a primary care practice managed by the faculty of Columbia University School of Nursing (CUSON), opened its doors in September 1997. CAPNA is the first faculty group practice in nursing with commercial, managed care contracts that reimburse advanced practice nurses at the same rate as physicians.

A leader with many "firsts" in clinical nursing practice, CUSON offered the nation's first master's degree in a clinical nursing specialty (nurse midwifery), and, in 1994, it initiated the first faculty-managed and staffed primary care facility where nurses have admitting privileges to a major medical center. In that same year, CAPNA became the first advanced practice nursing group with full board-of-director voting membership in a major medical center's physician managed care contracting organization. In 1996, it achieved designation as the World Health Organization's only Collaborative Center in Advanced Nursing Practice. It also received the Distinguished Practice Award for Leadership in Advanced Practice Nursing from the National Organization of Nurse Practitioner Faculties that same year.

Involved in scholarly practices in a variety of settings for over 12 years, the faculty also had practice management experience. The first independent practice site, the Center for Advanced Practice (CAP), was conceived in the Spring of 1993, at the request of the president of the Presbyterian Hospital.

CAP responded to the hospital's need to expand primary care sites serving the immediate community via its ambulatory care network. The practice presented an unusual opportunity to evaluate carefully the quality of independent nurse practitioner primary care compared with physician primary care. A randomized controlled trial was begun, and, to reduce variables in the comparison, admitting privileges for faculty nurse practitioners were granted on a two-year trial basis. At the end of the trial period, the Presbyterian Hospital's Medical Board adopted admitting privileges for faculty nurse practitioners as formal policy.

The science of primary care was increasingly validating cost, quality, and competence benefits of advanced practice nurses. Faculty reasoned that if nurse practitioner care is valuable for underserved populations, the same care would almost certainly benefit patients with less illness and more options for improving their health. They wanted the opportunity to demonstrate their abilities in a competitive market serving upscale consumers.

CUSON faculty at CAPNA have an average of over ten years' successful independent primary care practice, in addition to graduate degrees in primary care and national certification in their specialties. They are clinical faculty members with responsibilities for practice, education, and research. At CAPNA, their job is to provide comprehensive, high-quality primary care in the context of an academic practice under intense scrutiny, and, like all medical practices, to expand services in a tight financial environment.

CAPNA advanced practice nurses develop and implement individualized disease prevention strategies and health promotion interventions, empower patients to meet their own health care goals, provide health education to ensure optimal observation of health regimens, develop and implement plans for patients with chronic illnesses, and manage hospital care in collaboration with necessary specialty physicians. Patients' relationships with their nurse practitioners are enhanced through telephone follow-up. Careful scheduling ensures continuity of care. Whenever possible, patients choose to see their original provider.

The nursing school's long-standing relationship with the faculty of medicine facilitates development of carefully evaluated new programs for clinical care. The CAPNA venture was designed to build on this close alliance. Physician members of the faculty of medicine were asked to serve as advisors at many steps in the development process, and they contribute in the New York State legally defined role of physician collaborators with practicing nursing faculty. CAPNA's success brings new patients to the medical

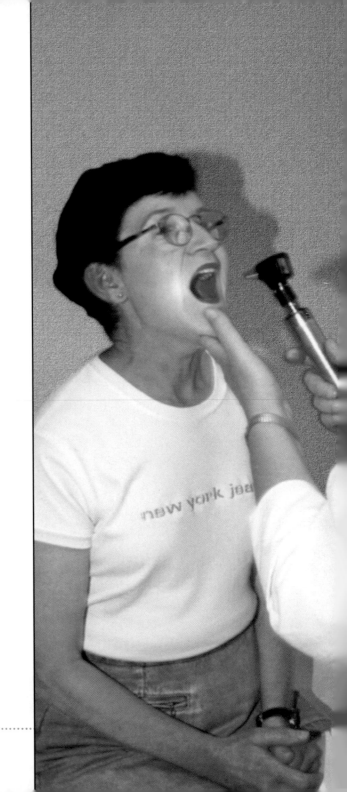

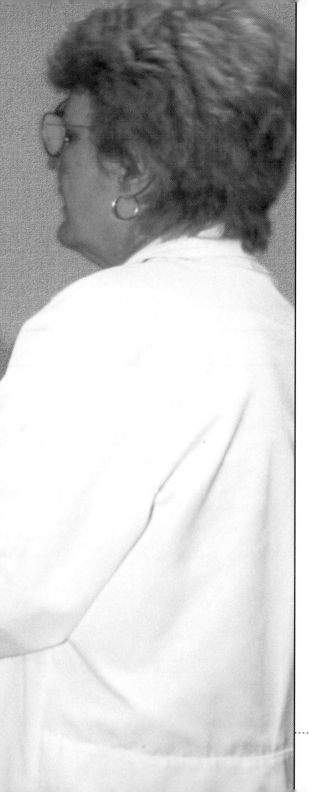

faculty. In nearly every case, patients—most of whom are new to the medical center—have accepted referrals to Columbia-Presbyterian physicians. Referrals are carefully monitored to ensure patient convenience and satisfaction, as well as compliance with managed care contractual requirements.

A scientific evaluation focusing on quality assessment and improvement is in testing phases at CAPNA. Patient satisfaction will be assessed in a variety of ways, and goals of the practice will be tracked to monitor progress. The evaluation will include a description of the demographic characteristics of CAPNA clientele and their reasons for choosing a nurse practitioner as primary care provider.

The business of health care is integral to the CAPNA practice. Funding was sought from supporters to do marketing research, demonstrate a target commercial population, and promote the new practice through a sophisticated marketing campaign. Initially, marketing efforts and managed care contracts were the prime sources for new patients.

Strategic alliances to promote CAPNA include representation of managed care organizations and other insurers' executive staffs on CUSON Advisory Boards. Provider-payer relationships are also seen as critical success factors at the operations level. Joint claims reviews, patient satisfaction surveys, and specific problem-solving initiatives are ongoing, and CAPNA management works closely with managed care medical departments to craft credentialing requirements for advanced practice nurses in the provider panels of the future.

Compliance with institutional and regulatory requirements is appreciated as essential by all CAPNA staff; internal alliances are solidified through CUSON faculty participation in medical center management groups developing and monitoring compliance guidelines. School public relations and development staff continuously seek positive media portrayals to promote CAPNA practice.

Nurses who accept the challenges and risks of serving new groups of patients have always advanced the profession and enhanced professional rewards for practitioners who followed. The professional commitment and accomplishments of the nursing pioneers who build the first highly visible independent practices like CAPNA, the trust of the patients who choose advanced practice nursing services and refer their families and friends, and the support of the nursing profession and health care community are all essential to promoting the role of advanced practice nurses and ensuring that their services will be available to increasing numbers of patients.

Advanced practice opportunities continued to unfold. Nurse practitioner (NP)–managed clinics and community health centers delivered cost-effective primary health care to thousands and research proved their worth.

In over 1,000 visits monthly, the homeless and needy get primary care from NPs at the center at UCLA.

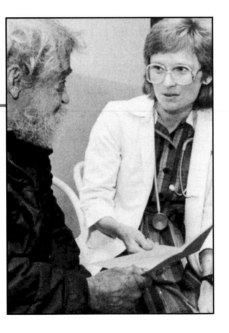

Nearly 800 babies were among the 2,000 patients who were treated in 1991 by six NPs and three RNs who staff the model Community Health Clinic in Lafayette, Indiana.

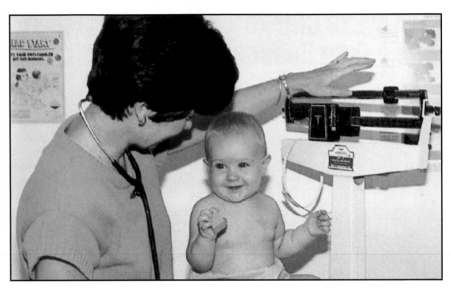

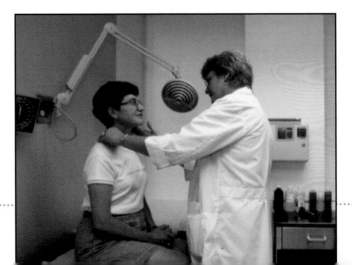

A $5 Day

It was a $5 day.
That's all I could say
to a person who thinks
a clinic like ours
surely gets its share
of the millions this country
spends on health care.
That's what our landlord thinks
when he raises the rent
and tells us he's pleased
to help us serve the community.
That's what the plumber thinks
as he works on the downstairs
toilet again and charges us more
than we charged him for a visit.
That's what salesmen think
when they call about high-tech
solutions and get-rich schemes
and what Trudy thinks
every time she pockets
the pHisoderm Soap on the sink
or loses the pills we give her.
But I know different.
At day's end when we lock up
the clinic and do the count
of patients and money and hide
the day's take in the lock box
under the desk in the lab
for Vern to deposit on Tuesday
I know different.
Sharon and I look at

the names of the twenty-odd
patients we saw today:
some new, some we know,
some young, some old,
some here, some at home.
We see what we did
and how much they paid
or didn't.
There's Tony, who's three
and not talking yet,
Ms. Stump, who can't stoop
to do the day's work because of
the nagging pain in her back, and
a nervous young man who gave
two names and thought he had
a social disease.
Dan Yeller's stomach was burning
like fire—he's the first to
admit he's back on booze
and Bonnie's desperate
to stop smoking crack for fear
of losing her job at the school.
Tonya cried when she found
she was pregnant. She can't
support another child.
Rosa was here, cradling
the fruit of her fortieth year,
a newborn boy—
and she'd been convinced
she could never conceive.
Two elderly ladies got

checked up for church camp
and Sateen Clark got
shots for school.
Miss Bea, who has sugar
and cholesterol, turns eighty
tomorrow in spite of it all.
Lula Hill we saw at home
to treat the ulcer
on her foot, and we made
a visit to Mr. Trim when
his wife phoned to say he'd
had another one of his spells.
Trudy arrived, to no one's
surprise, and lay spread-eagled
on the floor by way of getting
attention. Poor Ms. Gray
nearly suffered a stroke when
she opened the door and saw her.
"Well, my pressure's gonna be
up today," she warned.

These and others came
and went but no one came
with money. Not one check
arrived in the mail,
only a past-due utility bill.
The $40 we use
to make change was all we had
and we'd started with that
in the morning.

It's after six.
There's a knock at the door.
"Let's not answer it," I say.
"It can only mean trouble
this time of day. Maybe
it's Trudy back for more
soap or pills." I go anyway.
It's Tom, Ms. Carter's
oldest boy. "My mother
sent me to give you this.
She wants to pay something
on her bill. She said
for me to say thanks.
Thanks."
He's gone like a shot.
I close the door, open
the envelope and count
the five singles inside.
"Well," says Sharon,
writing it down,
"I thought today would
add up to nothing but now
it's a $5 day."

VENETA MASSON, DECEMBER 1992

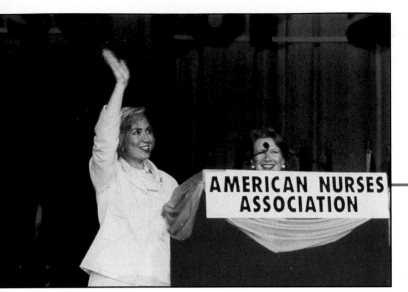

Rallying RNs at Massachusetts' state house, Boston College nursing professor Judith Shindul-Rothschild urges them to stand firm against staffing trends that undermine patient care. She surveyed 10,000 nurses about the quality of care in their workplaces.

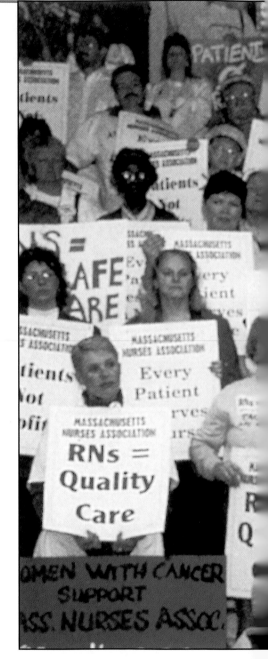

"America does not need half-baked, halfhearted reform," Hillary Clinton told ANA's 1994 convention. She predicted that job losses for RNs "will only get worse" if the system isn't changed. With her at the podium is ANA President Virginia Trotter Betts.

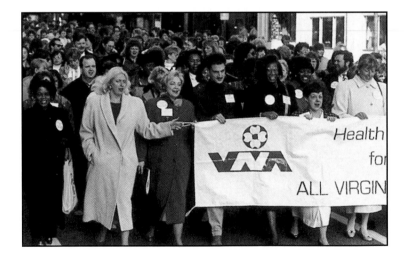

Over 1,000 RNs marched on the capitol in Richmond to show their support for "Health Care for All Virginians." The rally was led by the Virginia Nurses Association.

"*We* *don't need any more commissions, research institutions, or trend analyses to tell us something is terribly wrong with the U.S. health care system. When Rosa Parks refused to sit in the back of the bus, she didn't need any microanalyses of inequality in American society; she knew that what she was experiencing was racism, plain and simple, and she was not going to take it anymore. Well, nurses and doctors know just as clearly that the greed of corporate health care is squeezing humanity out of our health care system, and we're not going to take anymore either.*"

JUDITH SHINDUL-ROTHSCHILD
DECEMBER 1997

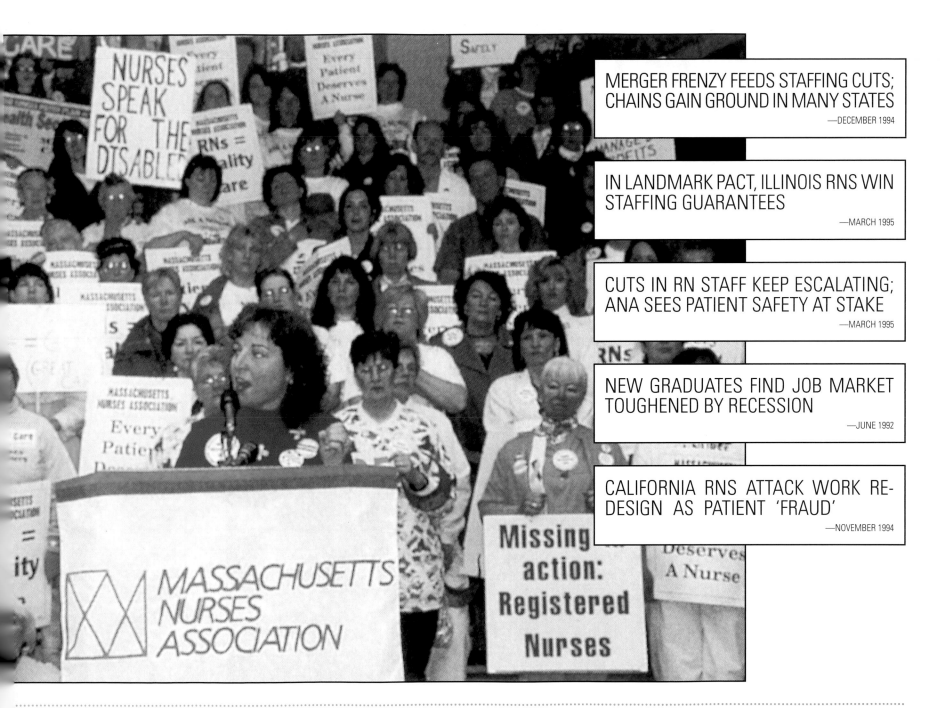

MERGER FRENZY FEEDS STAFFING CUTS; CHAINS GAIN GROUND IN MANY STATES
—DECEMBER 1994

IN LANDMARK PACT, ILLINOIS RNS WIN STAFFING GUARANTEES
—MARCH 1995

CUTS IN RN STAFF KEEP ESCALATING; ANA SEES PATIENT SAFETY AT STAKE
—MARCH 1995

NEW GRADUATES FIND JOB MARKET TOUGHENED BY RECESSION
—JUNE 1992

CALIFORNIA RNS ATTACK WORK RE-DESIGN AS PATIENT 'FRAUD'
—NOVEMBER 1994

Nurses served with distinction in Desert Storm . . .

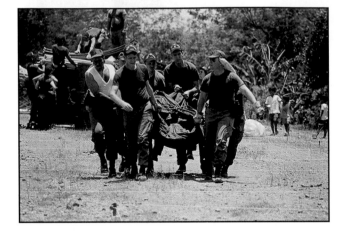

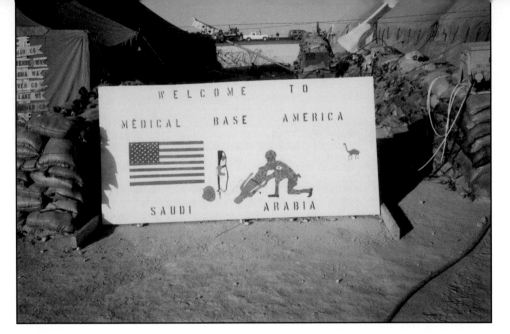

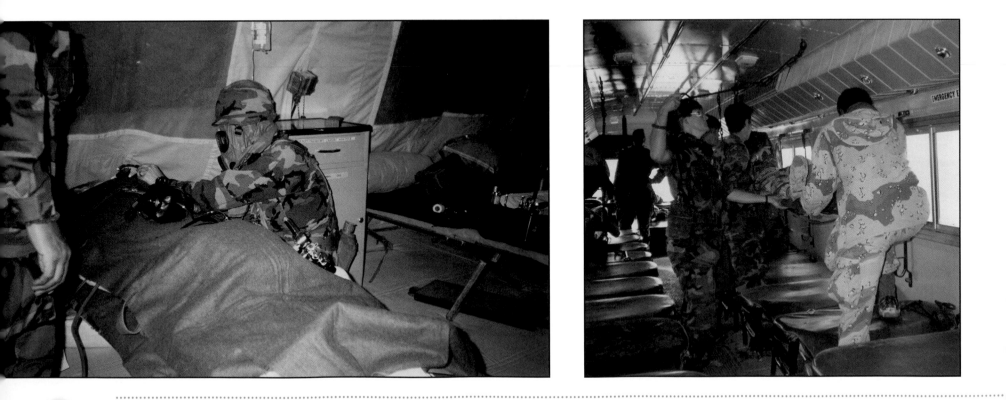

. . . and returned to hugs and cheers.

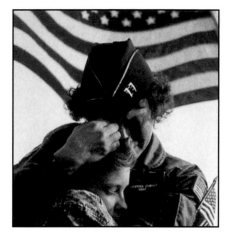

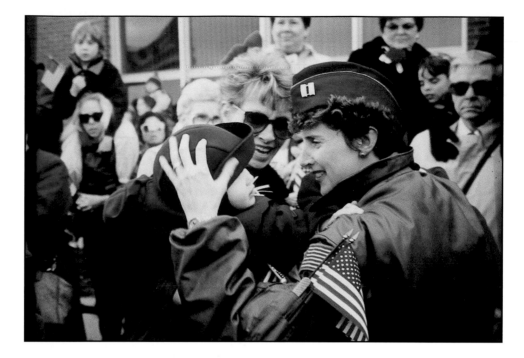

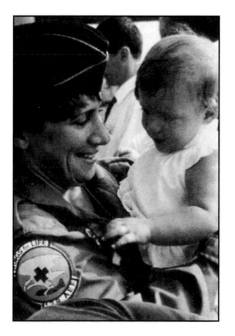

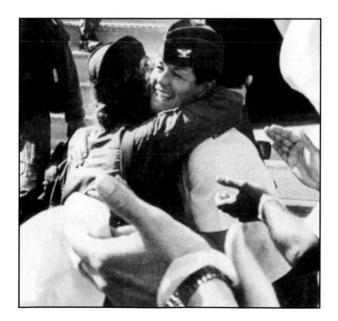

With her daughter holding the Bible, Shirley Chater was sworn in as Commissioner of the Social Security Administration by Health and Human Services Secretary Donna Shalala. Shalala had recommended her for her expertise in the health sciences and her accomplishments as president of Texas Woman's University.

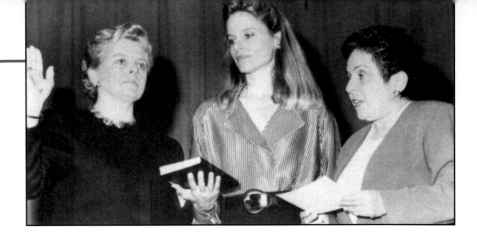

For her "personal courage," Colonel Margarethe Cammermeyer was ANA's choice for its Honorary Human Rights Award at a ceremony that was a highlight of its 1994 convention.

A decorated Vietnam veteran, Cammermeyer was discharged from her post as chief nurse in the Washington State National Guard after she was asked about her sexual orientation, and disclosed that she was gay, during a security clearance interview. In a case that made headlines for two years, she contested her dismissal and in June won a ruling from a federal judge, who said the military had violated her constitutional rights.

AUGUST 1994

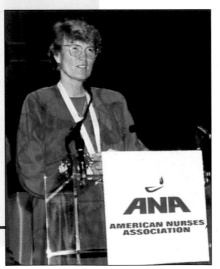

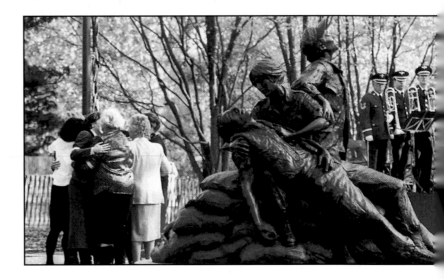

On Veteran's Day in 1993, nearly 20 years after the Vietnam War ended, thousands of military nurses and other female veterans paraded down Washington's Constitution Avenue on their way to dedicate a memorial to their wartime service. Donna-Marie Boulay and Diane Carlson Evans, former army nurses who served in Vietnam, launched the campaign in 1984 to pay tribute to the estimated 11,000 military women who had served in Vietnam. Ninety percent were nurses. Eight died in the line of duty.

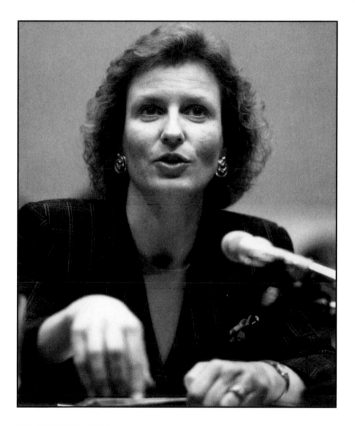

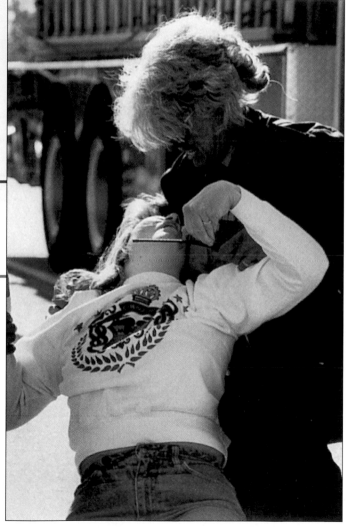

Weeks after the terrorist bombing that killed 147 adults and 19 children, nurses in Oklahoma City can't forget how the clock stopped for them at 9:02 AM on April 19, 1995.

Tony Lippe, a Sheriff's Dept. nurse, keeps having bad dreams about two-year-old Colton Smith, who died in his arms. For Bobby Johnson, a charge nurse at South Park Health Care Center, "it was just as bad as anything I'd ever witnessed in Vietnam."

Lives and routines were blown apart: "Almost everyone in this town was personally affected or is close to someone with a family member involved somehow," said public health nursing director Toni Frioux.

JUNE 1995

"She died doing what she loved," said rescue worker Sheila Hand, seen aiding LPN Rebecca Anderson as she collapsed after helping victims from the building during the Oklahoma City bombing. She was the only caregiver to die in the rescue effort.

Barbara Fassbinder, an Iowa emergency room nurse, was one of the first health care workers to contract AIDS. The 36-year-old nurse was infected in 1986, before Standard Precautions were generally observed. She spent the remaining years of her life lobbying and speaking out for protection for health care workers.

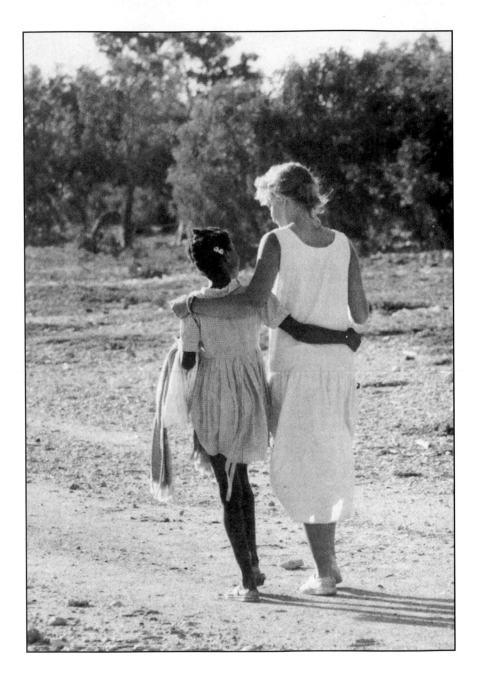

Despite the changes, new technology, the growth as well as the setbacks, at the close of the century, the essence of nursing has not changed . . .

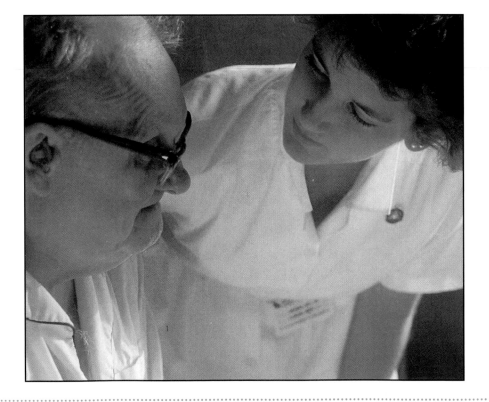

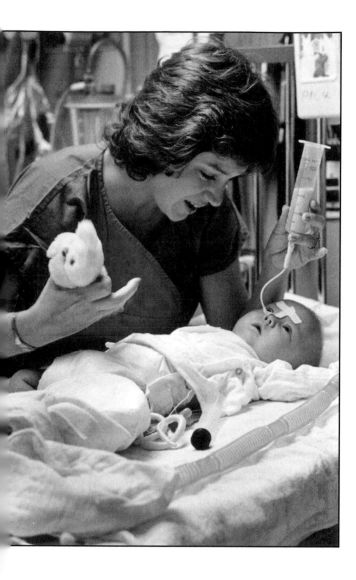

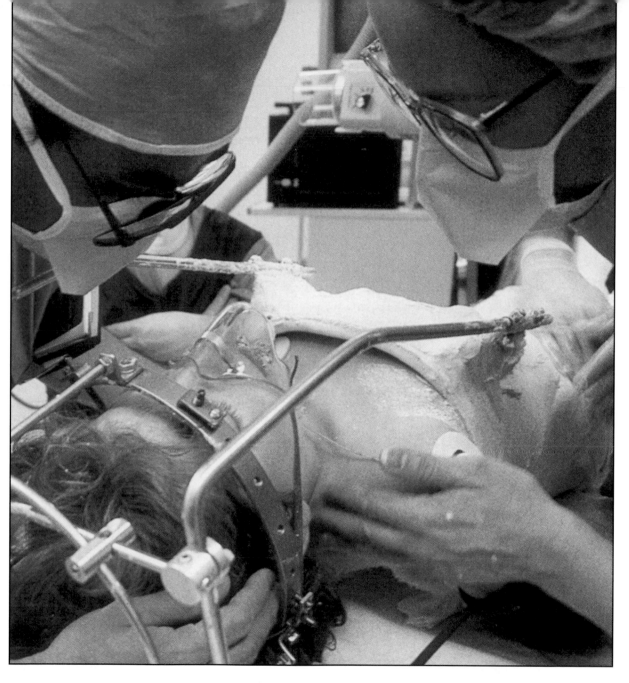

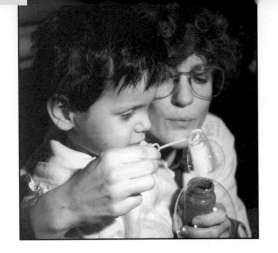

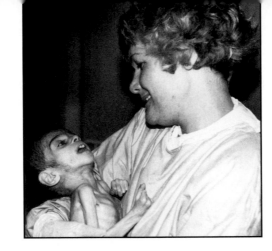

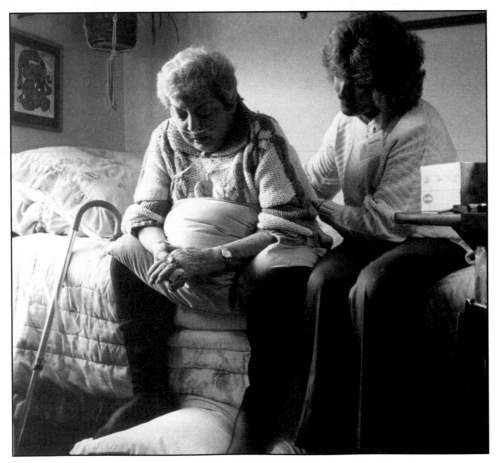

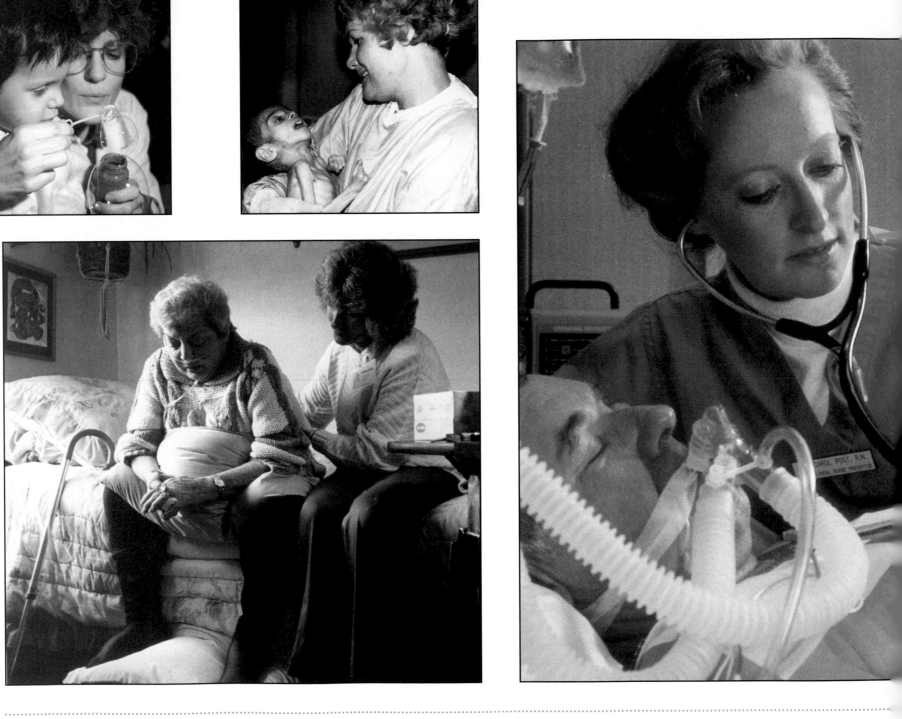

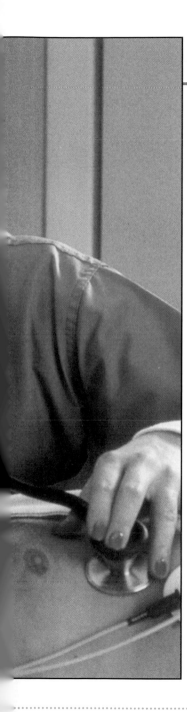

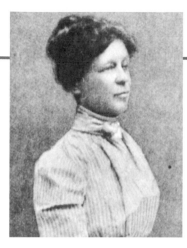

Commentary

Angela Barron McBride

Nurses, Nursing, and the Advancement of Women

Looking back on the twentieth century, one can argue that the advancement of women was a major theme, and that nurses as individuals and the nursing profession as a whole played a major role in that movement. Indeed, at least three interlocking claims can be made: (1) nurses played substantial roles in the century's key social developments; (2) nurses brought important sensibilities to scholarship about women and gender studies; and (3) nursing is the traditionally female profession that has most successfully transformed itself into a powerhouse field.

Key Social Developments

It is difficult to name a social movement in the twentieth century that did not involve nurses playing a significant role. Their influence was widespread, from Lillian Wald's founding of the United States Children's Bureau in 1912 through Florence Wald's founding of the Hospice Movement six decades later; from Rachel Robinson's work for equal rights and opportunities as head of the Jackie Robinson Foundation through Rebecca Rimel's work in support of volunteerism as head of the Pew Foundation.

Perhaps no individual shaped twentieth-century women's lives globally more than Margaret Sanger, the public health nurse whose experience in the tenements of New York City led to the founding of the American Birth Control League in 1922 and of the International Planned Parenthood Federation in 1948. Such advocacy for women's health issues was ably carried on by another nurse, Faye Wattleton, who served as president of the Planned Parenthood Federation of America from 1978 until 1992, and was succeeded by another nurse, Pamela Maraldo. In a real sense, the focus of this reproduction rights movement has been on the evolving staples of professional nursing: provision of services, public health education, health policy reform, and research.

Name an issue of concern to women, and nurses have been prominent in its development. Lavinia Lloyd Dock was a leader in the suffrage movement, then used insights gained in that context to point out how male dominance was the major problem confronting the nursing profession. Hildegard Peplau wrote eloquently about the therapeutic nature of interpersonal relations, and, in good feminist fashion, elevated everyday conversation into a powerful force for change with profound results. Wilma Scott Heide led the newly formed National Organization of Women from 1971 through 1974. Jo Ann Ashley was one of the first to explore links between paternalism and health care in the second phase of this century's women's movement. Diane Carlson Evans reminded everyone that women served in the military, and the resulting bronze statue of three women tending to a wounded soldier completed the circle of healing at the Vietnam Veterans Memorial. Shirley Chater's reorganization of the Social Security Administration in the 1990s resulted in the provision of award-winning customer services.

Women's Health Research

Nurses played a major role in moving women's health away from a focus on gynecology—synonymous with traditional reproductive matters—to GYN-ecology, meaning a focus on the fit between the woman and her environment. This shift is evident in the nurse's concern about a woman's dis-ease, and not just her diseases, and in the midwife's emphasis not on delivering the baby, but on how the woman wants to manage her labor and delivery. Nursing's ethic is a feminist ethic, concerned neither with merely "doing good" nor merely "doing unto others what one would wish for oneself," but with providing care that builds on the patient's perceptions of what is in her best interest.

Nursing's emphasis on women's lived experience has also had methodological consequences. Nurses have eschewed context-stripping techniques in favor of grounded-theory approaches. They were among the first to question a preference for the so-called objective view of the researcher over the subjective view of the patient, and to use diaries and health journals as ways to analyze the complexity of women's everyday lives. Nurses have also been concerned about the development of a feminist pedagogy, where the emphasis is on learning rather than on teaching.

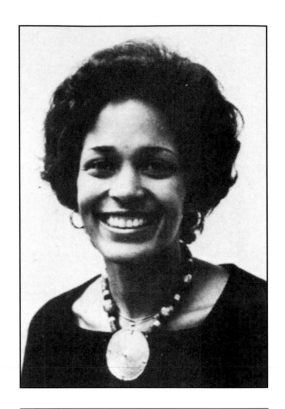

Faye Wattleton

The Transformation of a Traditional Profession

The advancement of women in the last century has been linked much more to women's having access to men's opportunities than to women's traditional strengths being accorded renewed respect. Indeed, the advancement of women has too often been equated with women not entering the traditional female professions, rather than those professions being held in higher esteem. One can, however, reasonably argue that nursing is the traditional female profession that has most successfully transformed itself into a powerhouse field. The aggregate number of nurses has reached record highs. Training is now based in higher education rather than in the apprenticeship model. Nurses increasingly have a career orientation that does not end when they become mothers, and is not limited to a concern about personal competence, but includes the expectation of mentoring subsequent generations and influencing not only the home setting, but health policy in general. Graduate education has moved beyond a functional concern with teaching and administration, to emphasize study of advanced practice. With the establishment of the National Institute of Nursing Research, caregiving research has become visible in new ways. A "doctorally prepared nurse" is treated less and less as an oxymoronic phrase.

Perhaps the area of greatest change is the extent to which nurses are being hired into positions that go beyond the discipline-specific and are not the province of any one field. Physicians and lawyers have long known that the MD and JD may be good preparation for a CEO position, government office, or university presidency. Nurses are increasingly being seen as candidates for such leadership positions without automatically being seen as "having left nursing." Rhetaugh Graves Dumas could be deputy director of the National Institute of Mental Health; Claire Fagin could serve as president of the University of Pennsylvania; Sheila Burke could be Bob Dole's chief of staff when he was Senate majority leader.

The twentieth century has underscored the extent to which gender is a social construction, reminding nurses of how gendered their profession has been historically with attendant negative consequences. These drawbacks persist, yet nursing has been more successful than any of the other traditional professions in moving beyond the discipline-specific to claim a broader mandate that is still linked to caregiving values. These gains have not yet been consolidated into broadly held new beliefs, but role models abound to point the way to the twenty-first century.

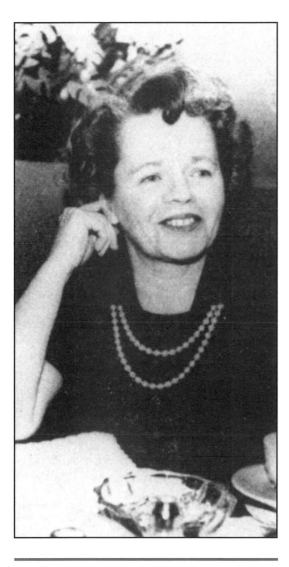

Wilma Scott Heide

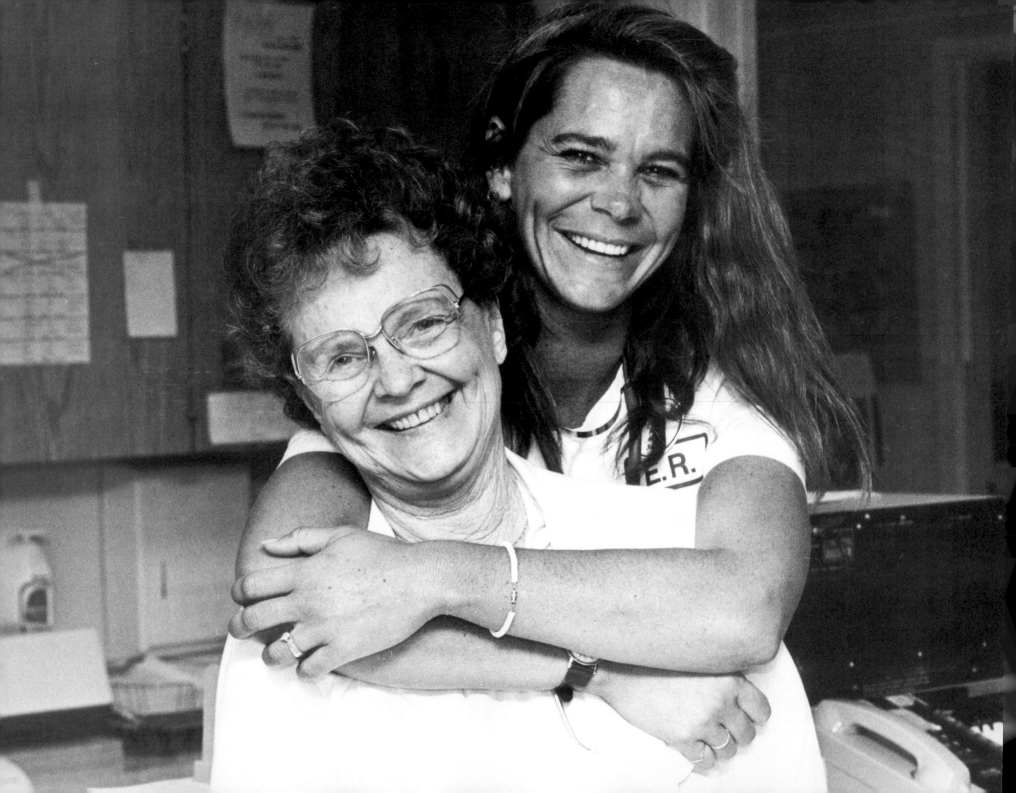

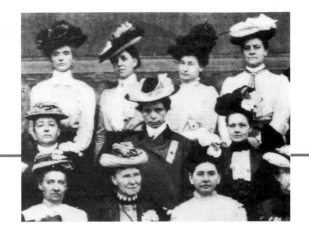

Faces of the Century

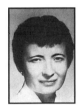

FAYE ABDELLAH
assistant surgeon general and
chief nurse, USPHS

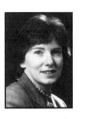

LINDA AIKEN
nurse-scientist,
researcher, educator;
University of Pennsylvania

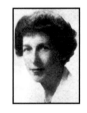

NINA ARGONDIZZO
nursing pioneer in
coronary care;
New York Hospital-Cornell
Medical Center

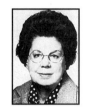

MARGARET ARNSTEIN
first chief of the Division of
Nursing, USPHS; dean,
Yale School of Nursing

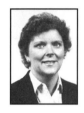

**MYRTLE KITCHELL
AYDELOTTE**
educator, administrator,
researcher; executive
director, ANA

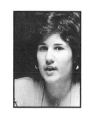

KAREN BALLARD
director of practice,
New York State Nurses
Association

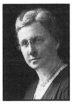

MARY BEARD
director of the Red Cross
Nursing Service and of the
Rockefeller Foundation's
nursing program;
recognized authority
on public health nursing

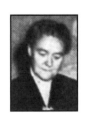

ELLA BEST
executive secretary,
American Nurses
Association, 1946–1958

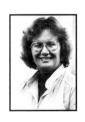

BARBARA BLAKENEY
public health advocate;
principal public health nurse,
Boston Homeless Services

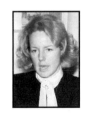

SHEILA BURKE
legislative strategist; served
as Senator Bob Dole's chief
of staff and as a dean at
Harvard's Kennedy School
of Government

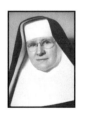

SISTER CHARLES MARIE
educator and ethicist; dean,
School of Nursing, Catholic
University of America

PAMELA CIPRIANO
administrator for clinical
services and chief nursing
officer, Medical University
of South Carolina;
past president of National
Student Nurses' Association

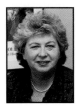

JOYCE CLIFFORD
renowned nurse
administrator; vice-
president–nursing at
Beth Israel Hospital, Boston

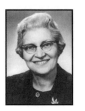

SIGNE S. COOPER
leader in continuing
education; chair,
Department of Nursing,
University Extension,
University of Wisconsin

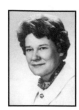

DOROTHY CORNELIUS
president, ANA, ICN;
executive director,
Ohio Nurses Association

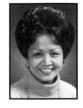

TITA CORPUZ
nursing executive on the
American Hospital
Association staff

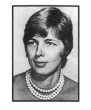

CAROLYNE DAVIS
first nurse to head a major
federal agency, Health Care
Financing Administration

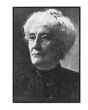

MARY E. P. DAVIS
first business manager, *AJN*,
and chair of the committee
that launched it

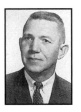

PHILIP DAY
nursing administrator;
president and publisher,
AJN Company

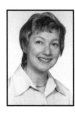

RHEBA DE TORNYAY
educator and dean,
School of Nursing,
University of Washington,
Seattle

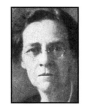

KATHARINE DE WITT
AJN managing
editor until 1932

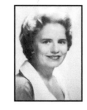

MARGARET DOLAN
public health educator;
president of ANA and
the American Public Health
Association

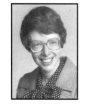

SISTER ROSEMARY DONLEY
educator, health policy
activist; executive
vice president, Catholic
University of America

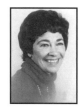

FLORENCE DOWNS
researcher, educator;
editor, *Nursing Research*

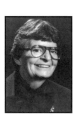

**KATHERINE DENSFORD
DREVES**
president, ANA;
vice president, ICN;
dean, University of
Minnesota School of
Nursing

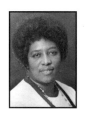

VERONICA DRISCOLL
spearheaded
economic progress;
executive secretary,
New York State
Nurses Association

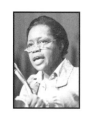

RHETAUGH DUMAS
deputy director,
National Institute
of Mental Health; dean,
University of Michigan
School of Nursing;
vice provost, University of
Michigan; president, NLN

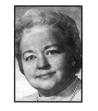

JO ELEANOR ELLIOTT
director, USPHS, Division of
Nursing; director,
Western Council
on Higher Education;
president, ANA

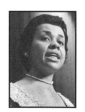

GERALDENE FELTON
educator, researcher; dean,
College of Nursing,
University of Iowa;
executive director,
NLN Accrediting
Commission

VERNICE FERGUSON
chief, NIH Clinical Center;
chief nurse,
Veteran Administration
nursing services;
president, Sigma Theta Tau
and American
Academy of Nursing

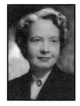

ANNA FILLMORE
first general director of NLN;
executive director,
Visiting Nurse Service of
New York

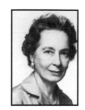

COL. JULIA FLIKKE
superintendent of the Army
Nurse Corps and the
first woman to become
a commissioned officer

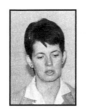

MARY FOLEY
first vice president, ANA;
director of nursing,
St. Francis Memorial,
San Francisco

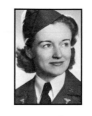

RUTH FREEMAN
noted public health nurse
and educator; professor at
Johns Hopkins School of
Hygiene and Public Health

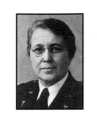

LT. RUTH M. GARDINER
first nurse killed in action
in World War II; an Army
Air Force hospital
is named for her

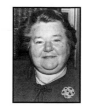

MARY ANN GARRIGAN
educator and
historian; curator,
Nursing Archives,
Boston University

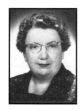

LUCY GERMAIN
nursing service administrator
and executive director,
AJN Company

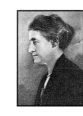

ANNIE W. GOODRICH
crusading educator; dean,
Army and Yale Schools of
Nursing; founding president
of the Association of
Collegiate Schools of
Nursing; president,
ANA, NLNE, ICN

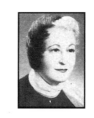

STELLA GOOSTRAY
principal,
School of Nursing,
Children's Hospital, Boston;
president, NLNE

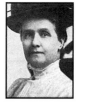

LYDIA E. HALL
nursing visionary; founding
director, Loeb Center for
Nursing and Rehabilitation,
Montefiore Hospital,
New York City

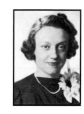

ESTHER VOORHEES HASSAN
first chief nurse, U.S. Navy

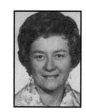

LULU WOLF
(LATER HASSENPLUG)
leader in nursing
education; dean,
UCLA School of Nursing

NELLIE X. HAWKINSON
professor of nursing
education, University of
Chicago; president, NLNE

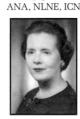

COL. INEZ HAYNES
chief, Army Nurse Corps;
general director, NLN

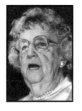

VIRGINIA HENDERSON
scholar, author, educator,
researcher; known
worldwide for her
definition of nursing

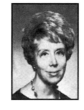

ADELE HERWITZ
executive, ANA;
executive director, ICN;
founding director,
Commission on Graduates of
Foreign Nursing Schools

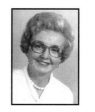

EILEEN JACOBI
educator, administrator;
executive director, ANA;
dean, Adelphi University and
University of Texas, El Paso
Schools of Nursing

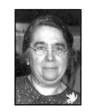

ADA JACOX
educator, researcher, health
policy expert; cochair,
Agency for Health Care
Policy and Research panel
that developed Clinical
Practice Guidelines for
Acute Pain Management

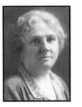

SALLY JOHNSON
principal, School of Nursing,
Massachusetts General
Hospital, Boston

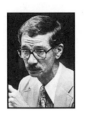

CLIFFORD JORDAN
educator, administrator;
executive director,
Association of Operating
Room Nurses

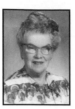

DOROTHY KELLY
editor, *Supervisor Nurse*
and *The Catholic Nurse*

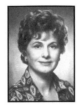

LUCIE KELLY
educator, administrator,
health policy adviser,
author; editor,
Nursing Outlook

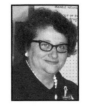

HARRIET BERGER KOCH
innovator, educator, author,
and founder of Video
Nursing; vice president,
AJN Company

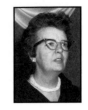

ELEANOR LAMBERTSEN
educator, administrator,
researcher, philosopher;
developed team nursing
concept

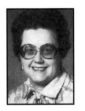

MADELEINE LEININGER
educator, theorist;
pioneer in
transcultural nursing

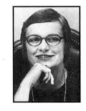

RUTH LUBIC
nurse-midwife,
administrator, innovator;
established birthing
center at New York's
Maternity Center Association;
recipient, McArthur
genius award of $350,000

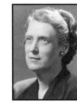

ANN MAGNUSSEN
national director,
American Red Cross Nursing
and Health Services

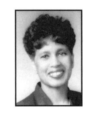

BEVERLY MALONE
president, ANA; professor,
North Carolina A&T State
University, Greensboro

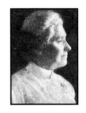

INGEBORG MAUKSCH
pioneering nurse
practitioner, educator,
entrepreneur

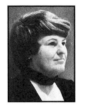

ANNA C. MAXWELL
founder of the Presbyterian
Hospital School of
Nursing in New York City;
Spanish-American
war heroine

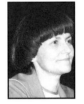

MARGARET MCCLURE
educator, administrator,
researcher; vice-president,
hospital operations,
New York University
Medical Center

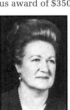

ERLINE MCGRIFF
educator and head of the
Division of Nursing at
New York University

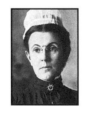

ISABEL MCISAAC
as interstate secretary did
field work for ANA, NLNE,
AJN and ARC; author,
educator, motivator;
superintendent, Illinois
Training School and
Army Nurse Corps

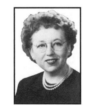

PEARL MCIVER
public health leader;
founder, U.S. Public Health
Nursing Service; served
two years as president,
AJN Company

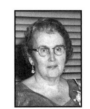

R. LOUISE MCMANUS
director of the
Division of Nursing,
Teachers College,
Columbia University

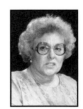

HELEN M. MIRAMONTES
educator and advocate for
AIDS education and
prevention programs;
member, President's Advisory
Council on AIDS; associate
professor at University of
California, San Francisco

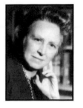

MILDRED MONTAG
professor, Teachers College,
Columbia University; did
original research on associate
degree program in
community colleges

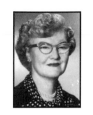

MARY KELLY MULLANE
visionary educator; dean,
College of Nursing,
University of Illinois

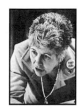

MARY MUNGER
chair, ANA Economic and
General Welfare Commission;
executive director, Montana
Nurses Association

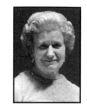

HELEN NAHM
first director of NLN's school
accreditation program; dean,
University of California,
San Francisco
School of Nursing

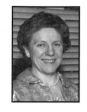

LUCILLE NOTTER
educator, researcher, author;
editor, *Nursing Research*

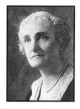

CLARA D. NOYES
director of nursing service
and chairman, National
Committee on American Red
Cross Nursing; president,
ANA, NLNE, and the
AJN Company

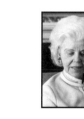

MARY ADELAIDE NUTTING
renowned educator, author,
scholar; first nurse to become
a professor at a university,
Teachers College,
Columbia University

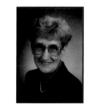

AGNES OHLSON
state board official;
president, ANA and ICN;
first president of American
Nurses Foundation

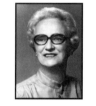

MARY ELLEN PATTON
staff nurse, Youngstown
(Ohio) Hospital Association;
in 1966, led 450 nurses in a
historic work stoppage that
received nationwide support

HILDEGARD PEPLAU
psychiatric nursing expert,
educator, author, theorist;
developed and published
interpersonal relations
theory; ANA executive
director and president

ELIZABETH K., PORTER
educator; president, ANA;
professor, Western Reserve;
lifelong fighter for
economic justice for nurses

ISABEL HAMPTON ROBB
visionary educator;
established Johns Hopkins
School for Nurses;
first ANA president and
also president of NLNE

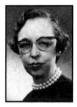

MARTHA ROGERS
educator, scholar, scientist;
head, Division of Nursing,
New York University;
developed the Science of
Unitary Man

ILDAURA MURILLO ROHDE
psychiatric nurse, educator;
president, National
Association of
Hispanic Nurses

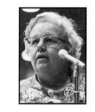

JUDITH YATES RYAN
executive director, ANA;
executive and fellow,
Lutheran General Health
Care Services

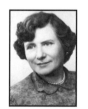

UNDINE SAMS
private duty nurse, articulate
spokesperson for private
duty and staff nurses

EMILIE SARGEANT
executive director,
Visiting Nurse Service of
Detroit, member of the
executive committee on
Distribution of Nursing
Services to assist in
recovery effort following
the depression

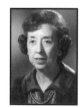

ROZELLA SCHLOTFELDT
nurse educator; dean, Frances
Payne Bolton School of
Nursing, Case Western
Reserve University; was a
pioneer in promoting
unification model

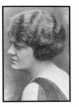

ALMA H. SCOTT
executive secretary,
ANA, 1933–1946

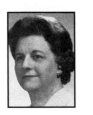

JESSIE M. SCOTT
director,
USPHS Division of Nursing;
staff, Pennsylvania
Nurses Association

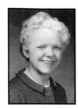

RUTH SLEEPER
director, Massachusetts
General Hospital; president,
NLNE and first president of
NLN after 1952
reorganization of nursing
organizations

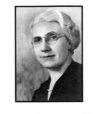

ELIZABETH STERLING SOULE
pioneering educator; director,
School of Nursing,
University of Washington,
Seattle; in 1931 established
Harborview Division as a
demonstration hospital
for nursing students

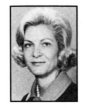

AUDREY SPECTOR
executive director,
Council on Collegiate
Education in Nursing, and
nursing programs director
for Southern Regional
Education Board

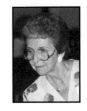

MARGARET STAFFORD
coronary care specialist,
Cook County Hospital,
Chicago and local unit leader

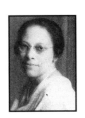

MABEL STAUPERS
first executive director and
last president of the National
Association of Colored
Graduate Nurses; authored
No Time for Prejudice

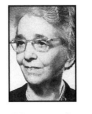

ISABEL MAITLAND STEWART
professor then director of the
nursing program at Teachers
College, Columbia
University; co-authored
NLNE's *Standard Curriculum
for Schools of Nursing*

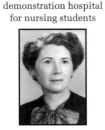

MAJOR JULIA STIMSON
superintendent of the Army
Nurse Corps and ANA president at outbreak of WWII;
also chaired National Nursing
Council for National Defense
and was dean of the Army
School of Nursing

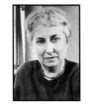

RUTH TAYLOR
public health nurse;
director of nursing services
for USPHS Children's
Bureau; nursing director,
International Health Division
of Rockefeller Foundation

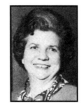

SHIRLEY TITUS
advocate for nurses economic
security; educator,
administrator, executive
director, California Nurses
Association; dean, Vanderbilt
University School of Nursing

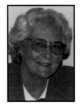

NELL WATTS
executive secretary,
Sigma Theta Tau
International

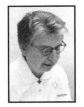

ERNESTINE WEIDENBACH
author, administrator,
maternal/infant nursing
expert; executive secretary
Nursing Information Bureau
(NIB), the profession's public
relations initiative from
1934 to 1948

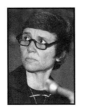

CATHRYNE WELCH
executive director,
Foundation of the New York
State Nurses Association
and Nurses House

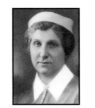

DOROTHY WHEELER
executive secretary,
New York City Nursing
Council for War Service;
director, Veterans
Administration Nursing
Service

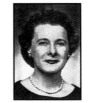

JUDITH G. WHITAKER
executive secretary, ANA

ANNA D. WOLF
director, School of Nursing
and Nursing Service at New
York Hospital; director, Johns
Hopkins Hospital School of
Nursing; established
University of Chicago Clinics
and also served as professor
of nursing at University
of Chicago

MARY WOODY
nursing service administrator
and educator, Grady
Memorial Hospital and
Emory University Hospital,
Atlanta; dean, Auburn
University School of Nursing;
chair, board of directors,
AJN Company

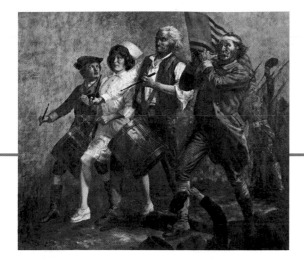

Commentators

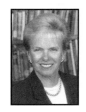

ELLEN D. BAER, PhD, RN, FAAN
historian and professor emeritus of nursing, University of Pennsylvania

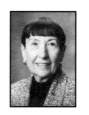

PATRICIA BENNER, PhD, RN, FAAN
professor, University of California-San Francisco School of Nursing; author, *From Novice to Expert*

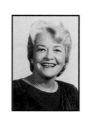

NETTIE BIRNBACH, EdD, RN, FAAN
president, American Association for the History of Nursing; professor emeritus, State University of New York Health Sciences Center College of Nursing

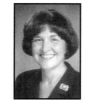

NANCY K. BOCCUZZI, MA, MPH, RN
associate dean for practice development, Columbia University School of Nursing

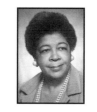

M. ELIZABETH CARNEGIE, DPA, RN, FAAN
former editor, *Nursing Research*; editor, educator, consultant in scientific writing and author of *The Path We Tread*

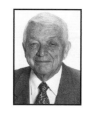

LUTHER CHRISTMAN, PhD, RN, FAAN
dean emeritus, College of Nursing, Rush-Presbyterian-St. Luke's Medical Center

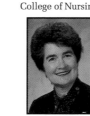

CLAIRE FAGIN, PhD, RN, FAAN
leadership professor and dean emeritus, University of Pennsylvania School of Nursing

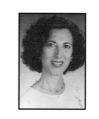

ADA SUE HINSHAW, PhD, RN, FAAN
dean, University of Michigan School of Nursing; former director, National Institute of Nursing Research

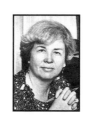

CONSTANCE HOLLERAN, MSN, RN, FAAN
senior fellow, University of Pennsylvania School of Nursing; former executive director, International Council of Nurses; former deputy director, ANA, government relations

DIANE J. MANCINO, EdD, RN, CAE
executive director, National Student Nurses Association

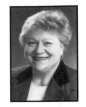

ANGELA BARRON McBRIDE, PhD, RN, FAAN
dean, Indiana University School of Nursing; author of several trade books including the highly successful *The Growth and Development of Mothers*

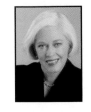

MARY MUNDINGER, DPH, RN, FAAN
centennial professor in health policy and dean, Columbia University School of Nursing; founder of CAPNA (Columbia Advanced Practice Nurse Associates)

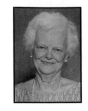

VIRGINIA M. OHLSON, PhD, RN, FAAN
professor emeritus, Department of Public Health Nursing, University of Illinois School of Nursing

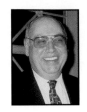

ROBERT PIEMONTE, EdD, RN, FAAN
former executive director, National Student Nurses Association and adjunct professor, New York University; former president, New York Society of Association Executives

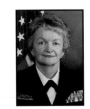

REAR ADMIRAL JULIA PLOTNICK, RN, FAAN
retired, U.S. Navy; former chief nurse and assistant surgeon general, USPHS; faculty at Rutgers University

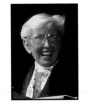

MARGRETTA MADDEN STYLES, EdD, RN, FAAN
professor and dean emeritus, University of California-San Francisco; former president, ANA; former president, ICN; immediate past president, American Nurses Credentialing Center

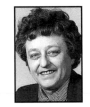

JEAN WOOD, PhD, RN
former director of nursing, Chicago Department of Health

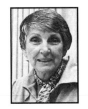

ANNE ZIMMERMAN, RN, FAAN
former president, ANA; former executive administrator, Illinois Nurses Association

Index

Photograph Credits

All photos not otherwise credited are taken from
the American Journal of Nursing *archives with permission.*

CHAPTER 1

P. 10: (*top*) New York Hospital, New York City; (*bottom*) St. Luke's Hospital, Chicago; p. 12: VNA Collection, Department of Special Collections, Boston University; p. 14: (*top left and bottom right*) VNA Collection, Department of Special Collections, Boston University; p. 15: American Red Cross; p. 16: VNA Collection, Department of Special Collections, Boston University

CHAPTER 2

P. 23: American Red Cross; p. 25: *(left)* Underwood and Underwood, New York; p. 26: Irene Kaufman Settlement Nursing Service; p. 27: American Red Cross; p. 28: (*all*) VNA Collection, Department of Special Collections, Boston University; pp. 30–31: American Red Cross; p. 32: (*top*) Underwood and Underwood, New York; p. 33: National Archives; p. 34: (*top left*) American Red Cross; (*bottom right*) Committee on Public Information, Washington, DC; p. 36: Courtesy of M. Elizabeth Carnegie; p. 37: (*all*) Hospital and Nursing Archive, University of Michigan; p. 43: (*all*) American Red Cross; p. 48: (*top center*) American Red Cross

CHAPTER 3

Pp. 51–52: American Red Cross; p. 53: (*top right*) American Red Cross; p. 54: (*left*) VNA Collection, Department of Special Collections, Boston University; (*right*) American Red Cross; p. 56: American Red Cross; pp. 60–61: (*all*) American Red Cross; p. 62: (*top*) American Red Cross; p. 64: American Red Cross; p. 65: (*left*) International News Photo; (*right*) American Red Cross; p. 66: American Red Cross

CHAPTER 4

P. 67: Wide World Photos; p. 69: U.S. Army Signal Corps; p. 70 (*all*) American Red Cross; p. 71: (*right*) U.S. Public Health Service; p. 72: (*top left*) International News Photo; (*top center*) Virginia de Carvalho; p. 73: (*top left*) Office of War Information; (*center*) War Relocation Authority; p. 74: (*top left*) American Red Cross; (*bottom center*) Photographic Laboratory, Massachusetts General Hospital; p. 75: (*top*) Acme Photo; (*bottom*) American Red Cross; p. 76: (*top left*) British Information Service; (*bottom left and right*) International News Photo; p. 77: (*top left*) Associated Press

Photo; (*top right*) U.S. Navy Recruiting Bureau; p. 78: (*left*) Press Association, Inc.; (*right*) Wide World Photos; p. 79: (*top left*) U.S. Navy; (*bottom left*) Official U.S. Army Air Force photo; (*bottom right*) U.S. Army; p. 80: (*top) Yank Magazine;* (*bottom*) Press Association, Inc.; p. 81: Press Association, Inc.; p. 82: (*top left and center, bottom center*) U.S. Army; p. 83: (*top left*) U.S. Army Air Force; (*bottom left*) U.S. Army Signal Corps; (*right*) Life Magazine © Time Warner, Inc.; p. 84: (*top left*) Press Association, Inc.; (*top right*) American Red Cross; (*bottom*) Glenn L. Martin Company; p. 85: (*left*) Official U.S. Navy photo; (*right*) Anne M. Goodrich; p. 86: (*left*) U.S. Army Signal Corps

CHAPTER 5

P. 92: (*all*) American Red Cross; p. 94: (*left, top right*) Esther Bubley; p. 95: Esther Bubley; p. 96: (*top left; right*) U.S. Army (ANC Collection); p. 99: (*left*) U.S. Army; (*right*) U.S. Navy; p. 100: (*bottom left*) Sylvian E. Ofiara; p. 101: Courtesy of M. Elizabeth Carnegie; p. 104: (*bottom right*) Frank Jones, Community Nursing Service, Winston-Salem, North Carolina; p. 106: (*bottom*) Liberty Flashlight Company

CHAPTER 6

P. 107: Esther Bubley; p. 109: (*all*) Peace Corps Photos; p. 111: (*top and bottom right*) Wide World Photos; p. 117: (*bottom left*) Robert Goldstein; (*top right*) NASA; p. 118: (*left*) Peter Dechert from *The Pennsylvania Gazette;* (*bottom center*) Bernard Cole; p. 121: (*top left and center*) Sandor Acs; (*bottom center*) Esther Bubley; p. 124: Dan

Bernstein; p. 125: (*bottom left*) Dan Bernstein; p. 127: (*top center*) Wide World Photos; (*middle center*) Sandor Acs; (*bottom center*) Arthur Davis; p. 128: (*bottom left*) Lankenau Hospital; (*right*) James Collison

CHAPTER 7

P. 129: (*top left*) Wide World Photos; (*screened background*) Lynn Pelham; p. 131: Guido Cassetta; p. 132: Wide World Photos; p. 133: (*bottom left*) Sandor Acs; p. 134: (*all*) Ann Dalton; p. 135: U.S. Army; p. 136: (*bottom left*) Marjorie Schorr; (*center right*) *New York Times;* p. 137: (*top left*) Sandor Acs; (*bottom left*) Reddish Associates; (*top right*) Staver & Scott Photography, Denver, Colorado; p. 138: (*top left*) Bill Emerson; (*bottom left*) Jane Chesnutt; (*top right*) Stanley Farrar; (*bottom right*) Arnold LeFevre; p. 140: (*top right*) *Washington Post;* (*bottom center*) Hank Young; p. 141: (*bottom right*) University of Maryland; p. 142: (*right*) Duane Garrett; p. 144: (*left*) Billy E. Barnes, Courtesy *Appalachia Magazine;* (*center*) Karen Gottstein, San Francisco; (*right*) Harvey Shaman; p. 145: (*top center*) U.S. Army; (*bottom center*) Harvey Shaman; p. 146: (*top left*) Bob Fitch; (*bottom center*) R. Summerfield; (*top right*) George Gibbons III; p. 147: (*top left*) John Pineda, *Tropic Magazine, Miami Herald;* (*bottom center*) Brooklyn Cumberland Medical Center; (*top right*) Gary Tassone; p. 148: (*left*) *San Francisco Chronicle;* (*top right*) Robert F. Lash, MD; (*bottom right*) Point Pleasant Hospital, New Jersey; p. 149: (*bottom*) Frank Ritter; p. 150: (*top left*) Peter Porter; (*bottom left*) Sandor Acs; p. 151: (*right*) *Scottsdale Daily Progress;* p. 151: Robert Goldstein

CHAPTER 8

P. 155: Christopher Gierlich; p. 156: (*left*) Terry Wild Studios; p. 157: Terry Wild Studios; p. 158: (*bottom left*) Jack Starr; (*bottom center*) Rose Lieberman; (*top right*) Sylvia Marquez, *UCLA Daily Bruin*; p. 160: (*top left and right*) Susan Bowser Associates; p. 162: Lynn Harty Siler, Henriette Egleston Hospital; p. 163: (*left*) Alan Zuckerman; p. 164: (*left*) Robert Belmar; p. 165: (*all*) Sandor Acs; p. 166: (*left*) Joyce Dinello; (*right*) James Kittle; p. 167: (*right*) Bill Binzen; p. 168: (*left*) Terry Wild Studios; (*bottom right*) Christopher Gierlich; p. 172: (*bottom left*) Christopher Gierlich; p. 173: Official White House photo; p. 174: (*top right*) Christopher Gierlich; p. 175: (*left*) Christopher Gierlich; (*right*) Terry Wild Studios; p. 177: (*top right*) Ted Mardin, Lenox Hill Hospital; (*bottom right*) William Thompson, *Vital Signs: Images of Nursing*, Addison-Wesley, 1984.

CHAPTER 9

P. 179: (*top left*) Richmond Newspapers; (*screened photo*) Jeroboam, Inc.; p. 184: (*top left*) Bill Burke/Impact Visuals; p. 185: Loyola University Medical Center; p. 188: (*center left*) Ascula Photo by Terry O'Donnell; p. 192: (*all*) U.S. Army; p. 193: (*top left*) U.S. Air Force; (*bottom left*) J.S.Carras/The Record; p. 194: (*center right*) Associated Press; p. 195: (*right*) *Daily Oklahoman*/Suba Photo; p. 196: (*left*) Bill Boyce; (*right*) Terry Wild Studios; p. 197: (*right*) Christopher Gierlich; p. 198: (*right*) The Image Bank/Gary Bistram; p. 202: *The Los Angeles Times*